No Fail Fat Burning for Women

Get the weight loss edge for your optimal physique.

BY

SKYE ST. JOHN

EDITED BY

LISA MECHAM

INTRODUCTION

Catchy book title, huh? Well, I had to get you to crack the cover somehow. Every word of the title is true. I'm proof. But before we begin, let's be straight with each other.

I know you're here because you desire a certain type of body; a certain level of wellbeing—whatever your definition of those things may be. There are other things you tried that briefly worked before you hit a wall or worse. It's important to understand that negative results aren't from a lack of willpower, but from a lack of solid, empirically scientific and proven research aimed _specifically at a woman's natural and unique biochemistry_. But let's go deeper because it's not only about fleeting and fluctuating things like scale numbers and aesthetics. What inspires your desires is emotion. You're _feeling_ something isn't right with your health and energy. Those feelings are strong enough to motivate you to _change your reality_. That's huge. You now have one point in the "Win" column by simply being here. Congratulations!

Now that we're on this journey together, let's both agree that you're the only one in charge of your reality. Your behavior and choices determine your success. That makes you an incredibly powerful woman. You are the CEO of You. Excuses have no place here. Check these things at the door: blame, self-sabotage and valuing the opinions of others over your positive growth and truth. You can be despairing or dynamic, but you can't be both. Having the initiative to get behind the wheel of your life is one of the most empowering actions a woman can take. It makes you a leader and role model. You have the right to be average but if you accepted mediocrity for yourself, you wouldn't be here.

When people talk about metabolism you hear the words "anabolic" and "catabolic" a lot. Simply put, anabolic means growth. Catabolic means destruction. Not only do these definitions apply to biological processes in your body, they also apply to how _you choose_ to experience your one ride on this big, blue marble. Growth or destruction? You are not your body. You are not your thoughts. You are not the opinions of toxic, unhealthy people around you who prefer misery for company. Osho wrote, "The mind is a beautiful servant, a dangerous master." When your mind takes over; when the "What Ifs" hijack your thoughts in the wee hours, feel free to take notice but don't attach. Don't be fooled. Thoughts are as temporary as storm clouds. You chose growth over destruction. You chose to earn a great reward _because you deserve it._

Ready? Let's do this. I'm right here if you need me:

Email: burnbodyfatforwomen@gmail.com
Twitter: SkyeStJohn
Instagram: Skye_St_John

CONTENTS

DISCLAIMER & ACKNOWLEDGMENTS

Very special thanks to my Editor, Lisa Mecham. An unparalleled writer, trusted confidant, a wizard of wit and insightful, unerring critical – yet compassionate — judgment.

Consult your doctor, priest, shaman, spirit animal or whoever you take your cues from before attempting anything in this book. The author and publisher expressly disclaim responsibility for any adverse effects that may result from using or applying the methods laid out in this book. You are responsible for your health and due diligence.
The information here is for educational purposes only.
Statements/products discussed have not been evaluated by the Food & Drug Administration (FDA) and are not intended to diagnose, treat, cure or prevent any disease or illness.
I have absolutely no affiliation with any of the people, products or companies I mention in this book. I only recommend what has worked for me in achieving optimum health. I receive no money from anyone or anything mentioned here.

Thank you to John Kiefer, Physicist and author of Carb Nite® Solution and Carb Back Loading™, Dave Asprey of The Bulletproof Executive™ and author of the forthcoming *Bulletproof Diet* book, Tim Ferris author of *The 4-Hour Body*, Jason Ferrugia author of *The Renegade Diet*, Tracy Reifkind "The Queen of The Kettlebell," and Dallas and Melissa Hartwig of The Whole 30® for providing the tools and roadmaps on my journey back to health and the physique I thought was impossible to achieve. Most of these ideas are not new but their research in taking them to the next level is.

Cover art by Angela Stucky Creative Designs
www.angelastucky.com

QUICK GUIDE

Commit to *at least* three weeks of No Fail Fat Burning. Most women find it so simple and easy it becomes second nature. Or, you can keep going until you reach your desired body fat, then Bulletproof® Intermittent Fast as your fitness levels require. This program is sustainable for the long term. For women like myself it's a no-brainer way of life.

What We Eat

- Fat Pg. 4, 23
- Proteins Pg. 22
- Vegetables Pg. 23
- Fruit Pg. 25
- Safe starches Pg. 24, 35
- Sweeteners Pg. 25, 26

What We Drink

- Butter Coffee Pg. 41

How We Eat & Drink

- Intermittent Fasting w/ butter coffee for breakfast 8am – 1pm Pg. 40, 56
- Break the fast. The 8 hour feeding window 1pm – 9pm Pg. 41, 56
- Days 1-10 Carb Depletion Pg. 54
- Carb reefed every three days after 10 day carb depletion Pg. 56
- Vitamins essential to women's health Pg. 58

When We Exercise

- Two times a week, no more than 20 mins Pg. 46

How We Exercise

- Choose from four short, fast, intense routines. Do two of them twice a week on carb reefed days Pg. 49

1 TO BURN FAT, EAT FAT
LOW CARB DOES NOT EQUAL HIGH PROTEIN

Guess what? I've got some great news. From here on out, fat is going to comprise over half your daily food consumption. No kidding. And it's going to be the best thing you ever did for your brain, belly and booty – among other things. Starvation to lose weight is sooooo 20th Century. And stupid. By following this program **I lost ten pounds my first week (typical), was never hungry** and have never re-gained the **15% body fat** I've lost so far. In fact, I'm still on the road to my healthy body fat goals while gaining lean muscle and increasing strength.

I've tried just about every "plan" out there but came to really admire the work and research of Dave Asprey of The Bulletproof® Diet and forthcoming Bulletproof® Diet Book; John Kiefer, author of *The Carb Nite™ Solution* and *Carb Backloading™*; Tim Ferriss author of *The 4-Hour Body™*; Dallas and Melissa Hartig authors of *The Whole 30™*, and Jason Ferrugia author of *The Renegade Diet*. Aside from some components of Dave Asprey's Bulletproof® Diet, the majority of information in these plans is geared towards men. The research and results on how these paleo-based principles impact women are scant. So many of the diets, exercise methods and research out there don't apply to women and/or don't take the gender-specific issues of women's health – and specifically hormonal responses – into account. Adrenal fatigue and killer cramps? Belly fat and bloat? It doesn't have to be that way. I am living proof.

I've pulled from these scientists, researchers and biohackers, testing what works on me and wrote it down here for you. None of the information presented here is a secret. It's just not what corporate food conglomerates, industrial agribusiness and mass media want the public to know.

My goal here is to get you informed and empowered about your health. You can reach your goals – permanently – and without the long trial, error and painstaking research it took me.

It's frustrating to read message boards or be in the gym hearing about great diet and fitness results men get. Women are starved for answers, proven research, results. Over and over you hear a woman ask, "Will this work for me?" Or, "I tried this and I gained weight. Help!" Unfortunately, most of the methods out there were never programmed with a woman in mind.

I've tweaked the methodologies of the biohackers I most admire towards a woman's unique biochemistry. I've had misses but now know the hits that allowed me to drop over thirty pounds, 15% bodyfat and still counting.

My hope is that you use this as a roadmap on your fitness journey and share the findings with your female friends and family. Everything that works for me as far as fat loss and muscle gain may not work for you, but simply try it for three weeks and, most importantly, *tune into your body*. It's the most intelligent machine there is.

My plan isn't only about looking good naked. Stay committed and that will come. This is really about turning your body into an environment of sustainable health. We're going to blunt the effects of internal inflammation, thus mitigating many life-threatening illnesses and disease. The best part. It's easy. No joke. This is easy.

What you need to accept before turning one more page, though, is that the majority of mainstream media health and nutrition information out there is false, dangerous, and making you sick and fat. You're about to learn the lies behind the food pyramid, typical American breakfast, whole grains, and the fear of fat. Butter will soon be your new BFF.

Counting calories is over. Eat the right proteins, fat, carbs at the right times, and your body will naturally adjust to a healthy weight and have you feeling like a ninja rock star. John Kiefer, a physicist and biohacker I greatly admire puts it best:

"Almost every single disease we have today is related to diet and too many carbohydrates too often."

On top of losing dangerous excess body fat, you can expect a lot of other conditions to alleviate or disappear all together. My adult acne (in the most embarrassing places) is gone and so are my allergy meds. I'll show you how I did it. If you want to skip the details and get down to nuts and bolts, head over to Chapter 7: Putting It All Together.

But first, check this out:

Summer 2013 family reunion. Two months before my fortieth birthday. My mom lives 3000 miles away so it had been about two years since I'd seen her. In those two years I managed to pack on over thirty pounds onto my five-foot-five frame and it was all in my gut, chest and inner thighs. Just like my father, I was a heart attack about to happen. He had his first massive one at forty and later a fatal one at 53.

I considered myself pretty active with a side of not-so-healthy habits: beer, wine, carbs, carbs, carbs, cheese, did I mention carbs? Oh, and a little more beer. I'm a former NCAA Division One athlete and an avid surfer, and Crossfitter with a black belt in TaeKwonDo. I also suffered crippling endometriosis and polycystic ovary syndrome after college. To be blunt, my menstrual cramps were like sitting on a chainsaw. My PMS cravings were insatiable. I had surgeries, every birth control pill on the market and even a medical menopause at 25. I followed the crappy Standard American Diet. Ate low fat, non-fat, avoided red meat, eggs. Ate whole grains, tofu, skim milk, soy milk, yogurt, margarine, beans. As I reached my late 30's my waist got wider the longer I ran, the "healthier" I ate, the harder I trained. WTF?

Fact: Muffin tops, FUPA's, love handles... whatever you want to call them. If you have a spare tire, that is your body's immune response to the food you're putting in your face. Just like any other medicine, food stimulates chemical changes in our bodies. What those changes are depends on food timing, quantity, and quality. You can absolutely control how food shapes your body on the inside and out.

But I digress. My mom sees me for the first time in two years and it's instant waterworks. But her tears weren't tears of joy. Her baby girl looked like a baby whale. I was swollen as a tick. The heaviest I'd ever been in my life at 150 pounds. I realize the number is relative. I have a tiny frame. For perspective, my normal weight before the gain was 115lbs. I couldn't get rings onto my fingers—or off. I understand weight is only a number and if you're carrying lean mass you're going to weigh more... although you will be much more fit and tighter. This wasn't my case. I was unhealthy, overweight and felt helpless to stop the downhill trend of my uphill battle. I tried juice fasts, veganism, raw food, vegetarianism. My mom is not one to criticize my weight or appearance (according to my girlfriends I really lucked out there). However, I know she was having flashbacks of my dad's heart attacks and could see it in my future. So could I.

I felt truly unattractive and sick. I live at the beach and hadn't worn a bathing suit in years. I didn't just have a muffin top, I had a bakers dozen. On a gorgeous, sunny Northern California day there was a street fair in my neighborhood. I walked home to change into a t-shirt and shorts. I couldn't fit into anything but an oversize sweatshirt and sweatpants. This wasn't just about the aesthetics. I felt helpless and hopeless. And since you're reading this, I have a feeling you can empathize. I stayed inside, threw a pity party for myself then decided I was done being a walking heart attack waiting to happen. But how? Everything else has failed or wasn't sustainable for the long term. Turns out when I was *truly* ready and committed, the answers came.

A friend who is a couple years older than me and an avid cyclist and surfer was dealing with some of the same issues. She lifted her shirt above the midriff one evening, exposing six pack abs you could grate cheese on. "Look!" she said. "There were abs under there all along." She said she'd been eating a paleo diet for a couple months. I had heard of the "caveman" diet but it sounded like another fad… and with all the butter, bacon and red meat they recommend, it sounded like a dangerous fad. But, there she was looking fitter, stronger, hotter, and healthier than I'd ever seen her. I decided I must go to there!

Based on my friend's recommendation, I bought *It Starts With Food* by Dallas and Melissa Hartwig. I committed to their one month Whole 30® nutritional reset challenge that provides the science behind the claims of eliminating or lessening a plethora of mental and physical ailments.

Note that I said they have the science to back up their methods. I'm not a blind faith person. My attempts at other dogmatic diets touted by the mainstream media made me a cynic at best and a bloated, depressed, heavier non-believer at worst. I want research and I want science-based results. *It Starts With Food* provides both. If you want the science and research behind these methods, buy the book. And, because I am a woman writing this for women specifically, I highly recommend you visit Stefani Ruper's blog at www.paleoforwomen.com. "Evolutionary health, Revolutionary Womanhood" is her mantra. Stefani is a godsend when it comes to a woman's biochemistry and what we can do to achieve optimum health. If you want to do a deep dive on research about why this all works, visit her site.

I became my own guinea pig; obsessed with biohacking my mind and body. What follows in this book is what worked to get me to my level of fitness today. Our biochemistry, health history, allergies, etc, are all different. Based on your unique set of circumstances, there are things you might want to alter once you've given my methods a shot.

If you have a working pancreas and do not use prescribed insulin, you can expect your body to respond positively to what I'm about to show you.

Here's all I ask: commit to AT LEAST three weeks. You can do anything for 21 days. It takes about three weeks for humans to develop new habits and routines that stick. Stay open-minded and listen to your body. When those three weeks end, you'll know what works for you and what doesn't. If you re-introduce dairy, for instance, and have a reaction, you'll know it's not in your body's best interest.

7

For me, writing this all down saves me from continuously repeating myself to my family and friends who want to how I made the metamorphosis happen. I have helped many of them drop unhealthy body fat and dissipate a lot of diet-related ailments. I hope I can help you, too. I understand the despair when you feel like nothing will work and that it's your fault. You feel like you weren't trying hard enough or didn't have enough willpower.

It took you a while to pack it on and it's going to take some time to burn it off. But it will burn off. When it does you'll have healed your body into making that fat loss permanent.

Fact: It's not about willpower or blame. It's about biochemistry, biology and what works FOR YOUR HEALTH and unique biological fingerprint. I was my own lab rat– with some expensive trial and error – so you don't have to be.

So, turn a deaf ear on the naysayers or people who tend to bring you down when you're doing something positive for yourself. Ignore the Internet trolls who spew ignorance faux-bravely from behind computer screens. The majority doesn't bother to research the science. I call them bumper sticker philosophers. They read headlines and assume to know the story. Beware of people who preach the food pyramid. It's a product of K Street special interests, politicians and foggy "bro" science.

Here's the cornerstone to reclaiming your health and physique:

To burn fat, you must eat fat. Namely, butter and MCT oil. Grass-fed butter. Not that low-fat, no-fat, margarine Frankenfood garbage. **Throw it out.**

WHY FAT MAKES YOU FIT:

Grassfed butter is rich in vitamins, minerals, anti-oxidants, and healthy fats. It's a nutritional silver bullet in burning body fat.

You must consume healthy dietary fat at higher levels in order to maintain muscle and keep hormones in a fat burning environment. When you say you want to lose weight, I assume you mean excess body fat. But a lot of people just want to see a scale number drop even if it means starving themselves and sacrificing muscle along with fat. This is called skinny fat and it's also the reason the lost weight returns plus some. I'm sure you've heard of otherwise "skinny" people having massive heart attacks and strokes. Skin and bones is not an indicator of wellbeing. Eating lots of healthy fats ensures your muscles are preserved while melting off body fat. Why do you want to preserve muscle? Besides the obvious aesthetic reasons, the lean muscle you gain and preserve determines your resting metabolism and your body's ability to burn body fat.

Starvation is stupid and dangerous. Skinny for the sake of an arbitrary scale number is 1. Not sexy; 2. A recipe for failure; and 3. An invitation to metabolic derangement and dangerous hormone disruption. Your yo-yo dieting days are over. What you'll learn here is so simple that there shouldn't be an overweight woman on the planet. Yes, it takes some time. After all, you didn't destroy your health and pack fat on over night. Don't expect to wake up tomorrow ready to wrestle alligators. It will come, though. Your body is a wise, sentient machine that always works towards healing in spite of how it's abused.

ALL ABOUT BUTTER

I eat over a pound of grass-fed butter and ghee (clarified butter) a week and have never been stronger or healthier. More about butter:

Source: Why Butter is Better www.deliciousobsessions.com/2012/03/butter-is-better-the-health-benefits-of-grass-fed-butter/

- Butter (grass-fed) is the best source of **conjugated linoleic acid (CLA), which has been shown to aid in weight loss and weight management**, as well as fight against carcinogens.

- Butter helps fat soluble vitamins be absorbed by the body

- Butter is a rich source of lauric acid (also found in breast milk and coconut oil)

- Butter is a great source of Vitamins A, D, E, K, and K2 (a great help with defeating PCOS)

- Butter contains Vitamin A, which is an antioxidant and is the most easily assimilable form of Vitamin A available. Vitamin A is crucial for the health of our thyroid, adrenals, and other organs, as well as absorption of calcium and proper development of children.

- Butter contains Vitamin D, which is vital for immune system strength and proper absorption of calcium.

- Butter contains Vitamin E, which is another antioxidant and helps protect our cardiovascular system.

- Butter contains Vitamin K which helps with blood clotting.

- Butter contains the elusive Activator X, aka Vitamin K2, which helps with bone strength and keeps calcium from depositing in places it shouldn't (like our cardiovascular system), as well as the proper growth and development of children.

- Butter contains glycospingolipids, which is a special type of fatty acid that helps fight gastro-intestinal infection, especially in children and elderly.

- Butter helps keep the joints lubricated and mobile.

- Butter is rich in short and medium chain fatty acids, which have been shown to ward against cancer and strengthen the immune system.

- Butter is a great source of selenium (if the cows feed on selenium-rich soil). Go grass fed!

- Butter contains lecithin, which helps with the proper assimilation and metabolism of cholesterol and other fats.

I'm lucky to live in California where access to grass-finished meats, sustainable seafood, and organic vegetables is practically everywhere. The most popular, widely accessible grass fed butter is Kerrygold Grass Fed Irish Butter. It's the one in the silver wrapper. My other favorite butters are:

- McClelland's Dairy Artisan Organic Butter: www.mcclellandsdairy.com

- Organic Pastures Raw Dairy (My favorite. They also sell/ship grass fed beef): www.organicpastures.com

OTHER AWESOME FATS YOU'LL EAT
- MCT (Medium Chain Triglyceride) oil
- Grassfed ghee (great for cooking along with grass fed butter)
- Coconut oil (great for cooking)
- Palm oil
- Olive oil (never for cooking! It has a low "smoke point." When it gets hot, the olive oil begins to decompose and the antioxidants in the oil are replaced by free radicals that damage your cells and are carcinogenic).
- Avocado

- Avocado oil (not for cooking. See above)
- Macadamia nut oil (not for cooking. See above)
- Grass fed, pastured bacon fat
- Grass fed red meat fat
- Pastured egg yolks

Make sure your animal fats are pastured, grass-fed and organic. If not, nix them. The fat in factory-farmed meats is loaded with toxins. You are what you eat eats. If grassfed meat isn't available, buy lean cuts and trim as much of the fat off as possible.

COOCOO FOR COCONUTS

What's the coconut craze about? Coconut has a little over 60% of a very healthy form of saturated fat called MCT's or medium-chain triglycerides. It's a shorter chain type of fat. Your body sends them straight to your liver, where they raise your metabolism and are burned as fuel instead of being stored as body fat. It's also an optimum brain food scientifically proven to enhance focus and cognitive function and has even been shown to help battle Alzheimer's. Pretty cool, huh?

MCT oil has shown great results in decreasing overall body fat and keeping it off. These medium chain fats also keep your body satiated longer. This is why they're so effective when combined with intermittent fasting. Butter contains a tiny amount of MCT. Palm kernel oil has a bit more. The king of sourcing MCT oil is the coconut.

The MCT oil on its own is flavorless so that's great for people who dislike coconut oil flavor. But, on occasions when I've run out of MCT oil, I always substitute coconut oil. MCT Oil is a prime fat burning fuel.

FATS TO AVOID

Omega-6 aka polyunsaturated fats (PUFAs) are not your friend. PUFAs create inflammation (read: disease, leaky gut and weight gain) in your body. PUFAs are:

- Nuts
- Seeds
- Nut and seed oils (except for macadamia nut oil)

Keep them to a bare minimum. I'll give you the full list in the next chapter. As Jason Ferrugia wisely states, "Treat nuts, seeds and fruit as you would condiments. Eat sparingly."

Try to avoid Canola oil at all cost. It's in practically everything, including restaurant food. Canola oil is an abbreviation for "Canadian Oil

Low Acid" and almost 100% of this oil is genetically modified by Monsanto. Canola oil is made from the rapeseed and used as an industrial oil. The modification process to make it edible for human consumption denatures its profile into becoming a hydrogenated oil.

Did you know Canola oil is illegal in infant formulas because it sabotages human growth? Moreover, the following conditions are linked to Canola oil:

- Abnormal blood platelets
- Free radical damage (free radicals are atoms, molecules, or ions with unpaired electrons that are highly reactive. In other words, they bind to molecules in your body, inactivating them resulting in chronic inflammation. All chronic diseases are just byproducts of increased free radical accumulation aka inflammation). Antioxidants help negate free radical damage.
- High cancer risk due to hydrogenation

From the Weston A. Price foundation and Fat Experts Sally Fallon and Mary Enig:

"Like all modern vegetable oils, canola oil goes through the process of refining, bleaching and degumming -all of which involve high temperatures or chemicals of questionable safety. And because canola oil is high in omega-3 fatty acids, which easily become rancid and foul-smelling when subjected to oxygen and high temperatures, it must be deodorized. The standard deodorization process removes a large portion of the omega-3 fatty acids by turning them into trans fatty acids. Although the Canadian government lists the trans content of canola at a minimal 0.2 percent, research at the University of Florida at Gainesville, found trans levels as high as 4.6 percent in commercial liquid oil. The consumer has no clue about the presence of trans fatty acids in canola oil because they are not listed on the label."

HOW DOES EATING FAT BURN FAT?

It sounds so counterintuitive to the BS the fat-phobic fear mongers feed us.

Our bodies regulate hormone secretion and enzyme production based on the tasty vittles we consume. If you eat more carbs than your body can burn, it's stored as glycogen (unused form of sugar) in your cells and that's why we sometimes feel bloated and pregnant with a food baby.

The other cool thing about fats like Medium Chain Triglycerides, Coconut Oil, etc, is that unlike other fats that take hours for your body to absorb, these little badasses absorb almost instantly and become available to your body as energy. Why is that awesome? Because if your body can access fat immediately, it will burn it. And now you're adapting and training your body to burn fat as fuel.

In *Obesity Research* and in the *International Journal of Obesity and Related Metabolic Disorders,* researchers proved that by simply adding MCT oil into the dietincreased fatty acid oxidation.

Their study, in essence, determined that eating fat burns fat. But wait, there's more. Additional studies also showed that eating a high fat diet along with lots of carbohydrates results in notable fat gain. So, it's not just about eating fat to burn fat. It's also about knowing when, how and why regarding carb intake.

Carbohydrates cause insulin release. Insulin has the gift of making body tissue grow. We want that tissue to be muscle. But in most of us it's fat.

Not to fret my fellow carb addicts! We're still going to eat carbs. Here's why:

After we initially stay off carbs for ten days, it is incredibly important for women to do a carb re feed about every three-to-four days. Especially if you're active and doing your short, intense workout routines, which you should be. You can't tone what isn't there.

If you stay super low carb for very long periods it will eventually slow your metabolism and cool off your fat burning furnace. By doing a carb re-feed, you keep that engine eating fat for fuel by "insuling spiking."

Insulin is a hormone released by the pancreas when carbohydrates (now converted to glucose) enter your bloodstream. It helps carry the glucose to either your fat cells or your muscles and liver. When you have excess carbohydrates (glycogen) in your body, your muscles and liver can no longer store them (aka insulin resistance) so guess where they go? Fat cells. That's why we deplete the glycogen stores by eating low carb and then spike the insulin with a carb re-feed after short, intense exercise when your muscles are the "hungriest" for carbs. The carbs now get stored in your muscles – instead of fat cells – helping the muscles grow and repair.

Also, carb re-feeds keep the mucus linings of your body from drying out. Moreover, it feeds the good bacteria in the gut. Don't go supersizing the French fries just yet. We're going to talk about which carbs belong in the re-feed in the next chapter.

Red Meat Myths

You've heard all the alarmist news about the dangers of red meat. They're true but with a caveat... red meat *is* inflammatory and toxic when it comes from factory farmed Franken-steer. Not only is the industrial beef empire inhumane to livestock, it's horrific for the environment and your body. Grassfed (and even better, grass finished) beef is literally a completely different animal that belongs in a healthy woman's diet.

Nine Reasons to Eat Grassfed Beef (Published by American Grass Fed Association c.2011)

According to a 2009 study (1) conducted by the USDA and Clemson University, grassfed beef is better for human health than grainfed beef in ten ways:

1. Lower in total fat
2. Higher in beta-carotene
3. Higher in vitamin E (alpha-tocopherol)
4. Higher in the B-vitamins thiamin and riboflavin
5. Higher in the minerals calcium, magnesium, and potassium
6. Higher in total omega-3s
7. Better ratio of omega-6 to omega-3 fatty acids (1.65 vs 4.84)
8. Higher in conjugated linoleic acid
9. Higher in vaccenic acid

What does that mean for women?

1. Lower in total fat

Cows were designed to eat grass, which means that they process it and maintain a healthy digestive system. Feedlot cattle eat a grain diet, mainly corn and soy, which makes for a quick weight gain and a higher percentage of fat in the tissue. Grainfed cattle also receive hormones in the diet, again to make them grow fast and gain weight quickly. This also results in a higher fat content in the muscle. Pasture-raised cattle are not given artificial hormones and so are naturally more lean than their feedlot counterparts. According to the Duckett study, the overall total fat content of pasture-raised cattle is usually about 25% lower than grainfed cattle.

2. Higher in beta-carotene

According to a California State University study (2), meat from pasture-fed steers contains a seven-fold higher concentration of beta-carotene than grain-fed animals. This is probably a result of the high beta-carotene content of fresh grasses as compared to cereal grains. Beta-carotenes are precursors of retinol (Vitamin A), a critical fat-soluble vitamin that is important for normal vision, wrinkle defense, bone growth, reproduction, and cell division. The overall integrity of skin and mucous membranes is maintained by vitamin A, creating a barrier to bacterial and viral infection. In addition, vitamin A is involved in the regulation of immune function by supporting the production and function of white blood cells.

3. Higher in vitamin E (alpha-tocopherol)

The meat from grassfed cattle is four times higher in vitamin E than meat from feedlot cattle and almost twice as high as meat from feedlot cattle that have been given vitamin E supplements.(3) In humans, vitamin E is linked with a lower risk of heart disease and cancer. Moreover, Vitamin E has been shown to reduce menstrual cramp pain. This potent antioxidant may also have anti-aging properties. Most American women are deficient in vitamin E.

4. Higher in the B-vitamins thiamin and riboflavin

Thiamine, also known as Vitamin B1, helps to maintain the body's energy supplies, coordinates the activity of nerves and muscles and supports proper heart function. Riboflavin, Vitamin B2, helps protect cells from oxygen damage, supports cellular energy production and helps to maintain the body's supply of other B vitamins.

5. Higher in the minerals calcium, magnesium and potassium

Calcium helps maintain healthy, strong bones; supports the proper functioning of nerves and muscles and helps blood to clot. Magnesium helps to relax nerves and muscles, builds and strengthens bones and keeps the blood circulating smoothly. Potassium helps to maintain the proper electrolyte and acid-base balance in the body and helps lower the risk for high blood pressure.

6. Higher in total Omega 3s

Like we just talked about, Omega 3 and Omega 6 fatty acids are polyunsaturated fats that play an important part in growth and metabolism. They can't be synthesized by the human body, so they have to come from our diet. Omega 3s reduce inflammation, lower the amount of serum cholesterol and triglycerides, prevent excess clotting and reduce the risk of cancer.

7. Better ratio of Omega 6 to Omega 3

More about Omega 6: While both Omega 3 and Omega 6 fatty acids are important individually, they also work in tandem and the ratio is critical. According to a 2008 study (4) a typical American diet can be excessively heavy on the Omega 6s – up to a 30:1 ratio – when the ideal is closer to 1:1. While the body requires some Omega 6, an excess can foster cardiovascular disease, cancer, and autoimmune disorders, which are suppressed by Omega 3s. The proper ratio can reduce the risk of those and other chronic illnesses.

8. Higher in conjugated linoleic acid (CLA)

CLA is another potent weapon in the arsenal against chronic disease. CLA can reduce cancer, high blood pressure, cardiovascular disease, osteoporosis and insulin resistance.

9. Higher in vaccenic acid

Vaccenic acid is a transfat that occurs naturally in ruminant animals, but unlike its synthetically-produced cousins, is important for good health. A recent study (5) published in The Journal of Nutrition showed that vaccenic acid protects against atherosclerosis, a contributing factor in cardiovascular disease.

1 S. K. Duckett, et al. "Effects of winter stocker growth rate and finishing system on: III. Tissue proximate, fatty acid, vitamin, and cholesterol content." Journal of Animal Science. June 5, 2009, doi: 10.2527/jas.2009-1850.
2 C.A. Daley, et al. "A review of fatty acid profiles and antioxidant content in grass-fed and grain-fed beef." Nutrition Journal 2010, 9:10
3 Smith, G.C. "Dietary supplementation of vitamin E to cattle to improve shelf life and case life of beef for domestic and international markets." Colorado State University, Fort Collins, Colorado 80523-1171
4 Simopoulos AP. "The importance of the omega-6/omega-3 fatty acid ratio in cardiovascular disease and other chronic diseases." Experimental Biology and Medicine. 2008 Jun;233(6):674-88.
5 Adam L. Lock, et al. "Butter Naturally Enriched in Conjugated Linoleic Acid and Vaccenic Acid Alters Tissue Fatty Acids and Improves the Plasma Lipoprotein Profile in Cholesterol-Fed Hamsters." J. Nutr. August 2005 135: 1934-1939

Everything Estrogen

Women with high percentages of body fat (25%+) have higher estrogen levels and insulin resistance that takes your hormonal balance, kicks it down the stairs and then stomps it on the curb. Carrying excess body fat severely stresses your body. It literally forces your system to rage against itself trying to burn the fat, throwing your hormones and metabolic responses into further chaos. Excess bodyfat also makes it hard to gain the lean muscle a woman's body requires to maintain healthy bone density and permanent fat loss. Building lean muscle not only makes you strong, fit, and tight, it also allows you to withstand the occasional overeating without weight gain.

If you're one of those women who shrieks, "Ew! I don't want to bulk up," you are mistaken. Unless you're on steroids, you're not going to bulk up. You need to exercise intensely for short bursts at least twice a week. We don't have enough testosterone in our bodies to bulk up without injecting ourselves with something illegal.

Men and women both have testosterone and estrogen in their systems. Women have significantly less testosterone, hence more fat and less lean mass. However, we need that all that testosterone to burn fat and maintain muscle. Due to environmental toxins, plastics, factory farmed meats, polluted oceans, and misinformed diet and exercise, most American men AND women have too little testosterone and too much estrogen. Man boobs? Check. Little girls hitting puberty at seven? Check. Fat deposits that don't disappear no matter what? Check.

Alcohol and Estrogen

Your liver is your body's filter for all the toxins (topical or ingested) that enter your system. For a lot of us, our livers become so saturated with toxins that we cripple its ability to metabolize fat. Moreover, your liver is constantly working to eliminate the excess estrogen in your body. Alcohol raises estrogen levels. If you consume it regularly along with an inflammatory diet, your poor ol' liver can never cleanse you of the excess estrogen and it cannot burn fat for you properly. To be blunt: every alcoholic drink you consume is a choice to hold onto body fat regardless of the other healthy choices you make. If eliminating alcohol for the majority of the time is not an option for you, this plan will give you mediocre to non-existent results.

Maybe you're still in the "wish" phase for a better body and not in the "willing to work for it" phase. That's ok. Set it down and come back when you're serious.

Like I said: I'm not into making pie-in-the-sky statements. As women, we get bamboozled enough with weight loss gimmicks. This is about burning fat, feeling superhuman, detoxing, and creating the healthy physique your body was born to have.

Ready? Meet me on the next page.

2 SCREW THE SCALE & EAT YOUR ASS OFF
FOODS THAT IGNITE A BLUBBER INFERNO

The idea of "calories in, calories out" is dead as disco. It doesn't take into consideration so many other chronic conditions that contribute to weight gain that most women are unaware they're experiencing. This includes, but is not limited to: insulin resistance, hormonal imbalance, leaky gut syndrome, and gut dysbiosis. Basically, when your gut is unhealthy from a diet of highly inflammatory foods (Omega 6's, gluten, grains, legumes, dairy, sugar, soy, processed Frankenfood) it severely impairs your body's ability to absorb the healthy nutrients you ingest. Thus resulting in GI pain, gas and bloating. Almost 80% of your immune system is in the gut. Unhealthy gut = unhealthy you. On the inside and out. Unhealthy skin is a sign there's something wrong. It's your body's biggest organ and billboard for your health. For a detailed but easily understandable explanation on gut health, disease and weight gain, check out Chapter Six of *It Starts With Food*.

Moreover, "calories in, calories out" is unhelpful if you are someone who struggles with hormone imbalance, PCOS, endometriosis, painful periods, adrenal fatigue. On and on.

THE SCALE
Screw it. Numbers don't mean much. Did you poop this morning? Well, there's a couple pounds lost. Did you NOT poop this morning? There's a couple pounds you're still hauling around. Where are you in your menstrual cycle? Did you drink a bunch of water or shower before weighing? That will cause flux in the scale numbers. So will weighing yourself at different times of the day.

Becoming obsessed with the scale is only going to be a dangerous mind game. It's going to be you screwing you. My weight doesn't matter to me as much as body fat percentage anyway because I know I'm gaining lean muscle mass. It weighs more but burns more fat even in a sedentary state. Google "five pounds of fat, five pounds of muscle." Go ahead. I'll wait. (checks email, Instagram, tweets.)

Oh, you're back? The five pound muscle is much smaller than the fat yet they weigh the same. You want more muscle. And no, you won't turn into

SheHulk. You'll be toned, shapely and strong. When I first started on this journey I resisted the urge to weigh myself daily and let my clothes and the mirror be my scale. However, once a week I used an Omron body fat analyzer and digital scale to track my progress. The Omron isn't the most accurate but it is consistent. Nowadays I take measurements monthly. I can feel where my body is as far as fat, bloat or muscle. The most important thing is that I'm healthy again and am proud of how I look and feel.

Here's how I measured my progress in the beginning:

- Once a week **at most**. At the same time, on the same day. Immediately upon waking **do not** consume any liquids and do not shower.

- Pee (and poop if you can). If not, give yourself a couple pounds leeway. Measure your body fat (and weigh yourself if that's your only option).

- Take front, side, back photos. It's always cool to watch your body morph into the physique you want. Things shrink here, things lift there. Plus, it keeps you going on those difficult days. Yes, those days will happen. But you're tough. You're gonna make it after all.

- Write your numbers down in your iPhone notes app or journal. Keep a note of the date and time with your photos. I also used to write whether I was PMS-ing or had done a carb re-feed the night before. That's going to change the scale number for a lot of people, but it **does not** mean you are gaining fat. Are we clear on that? Shake your head "yes." Ok. Moving forward. Walk with me.

WHAT TO EXPECT

Sometimes people see the scale number rise after a few weeks of losing pounds. That triggers a downward shame spiral of feeling like a failure or that all is lost although they did everything right. And then they go on an emotional eating binge sponsored by Nabisco and Haagen Dazs (or Pizza Hut and Anheuser Busch if it's me). There have been plenty of times my scale numbers went up but my body fat went down. That's a positive thing. So, get a bodyfat test and don't take the scale so seriously. In the beginning you will experience a good bit of overall weight loss (depending on how much body fat you have to lose and how much water weight you're holding). Then, you will plateau. Then, as you keep at it – because you will.

Don't make me come over there – As you keep at it, fat will start falling off randomly in chunks.

On days after carb re-feeds you will probably see a gain of a few pounds. Do not fret. It means nothing. Again, give yourself about five-to-eight pounds wiggle room during PMS and your period if those tend to be difficult. My horrific periods, mood swings and cramps have withered away to a three-day menstrual cycle I can clock with a stopwatch.

Other things to expect: increased energy, focus. Much less bloat and brain fog. Clearer skin, deeper sleep, better sex, and clothes that aren't as tight as they used to be.

HUNGER & CRAVINGS

The good news: eating an anti-inflammatory diet full of healthy fats is going to curb your cravings for whatever your gnarly poison is. For women these tend to be sugar, diet sodas, fruit juices, alcohol, dairy, bread, pasta, you know what you like that's no good. But it's not going to be instant. Craving is a mental, emotional want; not a necessity. Hunger is that primal need to fuel your body with nutrients. You should never feel like you're starving. If you do, add more fat and veggies to your meals. Speaking of meals…

HERE'S WHAT WE'LL EAT

First, we eliminate alcohol, dairy (sans grass-fed butter), gluten, most grains, legumes, corn, very starchy vegetables (mostly white potatoes), predator fish, sugar, most fruits, minimal seeds, and nuts. I tried adding dairy back into my diet with raw milk and raw cream. Immediately my allergies and acne flared up. Off dairy now for good.

If you read Tim Ferris' *4- Hour Body* he talks about a "Minimun Effective Dose" (MED) Theory. It is the smallest dose of something that will produce a desired outcome. He writes:

"In biological systems, exceeding your MED can freeze progress for weeks, even months.

In the context of body re-design, there are two fundamental MEDs to keep in mind:

To remove stored fat ➔ *do the least necessary to trigger a fat loss cascade of specific hormones.*

To add muscle in small or large quantities ➔ *do the least necessary to trigger local (specific muscles) and systemic (hormonal) growth mechanisms.*

Knocking over the dominos that trigger both of these events takes surprisingly little. Don't complicate them."

For example, if working out only 15 minutes twice a week can trigger lean muscle gain and fat loss, why would you kill yourself (and your adrenal glands) five hours a week doing chronic cardio and God knows what else in a gym? More on that later. But MED applies in your diet, too.

You need to experiment and work with what's going to keep you on track for most of the time with the minimal effective dose. Tim Ferris' "Slow Carb" diet didn't work as well for me as the Bulletproof® paleo variation combined with my own tweaked version based loosely on Carb Nite®. But it does for others. My "Whole 30" commitment of eating clean with mainly Paleo principles included intermittent fasting with butter coffee, carb re-feeds and only a week of the Rapid Fat Loss Protocol by Dave Asprey (it's all I could take). Ultimately, you know your body best. You are responsible for knowing what works for your unique biology. There are many paths to the same destination. If someone starts spouting dogma about "their way or the highway," raise an eyebrow and run away.

I'm sharing what finally worked for me and for many others (including my friends and family) after a very frustrating and rapid weight gain. Again, I'm not about fads or selling products. I'm about science.

For example, I eat chicken and other poultry because I have access to probably some of the cleanest and most humanely-raised meat in the world. Dave Asprey frowns upon it for his own valid reasons, but I eat it. There you go. Also, I very rarely eat fruits. Maybe a handful of berries in a protein smoothie. Dave Asprey allows for a few fruits in The Bulletproof® Diet but refers to most fruits as "watery bags of candy." Sugar is sugar. Fruit contains sugar. Some fruits more than others. If you have excess flab hanging off of places, then you, too, have consumed too much sugar in the wrong ways whether in the form of starches, grains, alcohol, legumes, or sweets.

Tim Ferris allows for more grains, dairy and a "pig out" weekly junk food day. Same with John Kiefer. Nope. I don't do that. For me, it's the equivalent of quitting smoking six days a week and sucking down as much cancer on the seventh. This might work for men, but for women this is going to cause metabolic derangement. Our carb re-feeds are going to stay clean because I'm not about causing insulin spikes with toxic foods for fat loss. I'm talking about consistently making healthy choices and not supporting the industries that have caused this obesity epidemic in the first place.

Cheats every now and again are human. We have remedies for that in Chapter Nine. The whole "everything in moderation" mantra makes me roll my eyes. Crap in moderation is still crap. What I'm saying is take what works for you and **your best health**, then stick to it most of the time, as much as you can. Special allowances for very special occasions.

Caveat: I do not consider our curves "flab." Curvy women – and women of all sizes and shapes – are perfect exactly as they are. They are sexy as hell. I'm talking about disease-causing fat from toxic foods and environmental pollution we're not biologically made to tolerate. What's causing all the heart disease, chronic inflammation and killing millions IS NOT dietary fat intake but excessive consumption of (and addiction to) carbohydrates, especially the refined ones.

I could care less about skinny. I want you – and me – to be healthy so we can achieve total world domination. Below is what we eat to get there.

PROTEIN

- Organic, Grass-fed Whey
- Organic, Grass-Fed Collagen Protein
- Grass-fed beef (grass-finished better)
- Grass-fed buffalo (grass-finished better)/wild game
- Grass-fed lamb (grass-finished better)
- Free-range organic pastured eggs
- Free-range organic poultry
- Organic pastured pork (including sugar free bacon. Do not eat factory farmed bacon). Remember that toxins store in fat.
- Wild-caught sustainable seafood
- Low-mercury fish (anchovies, haddock, petrale, sole, sardines, sockeye salmon, summer flounder, trout)

Fact: You are what you eat, eats. Grass-fed means the animal has been fed grass for most of its life but spent probably the last month (and a lot of times more) eating a grain (possibly gluten) diet. Grass-finished means it's eaten as nature intended its whole life. I realize these meats are much more expensive so if you don't have access to these meats, then buy leaner cuts and trim the fat. If you can access the clean meats, the fat on them is your friend. And soy, tempeh, seitan are **absolutely out,** especially for women. Why no soy? It contains isoflavones which are a kind of phytoestrogen that female AND male bodies recognize as estrogen. Unless you are peri-menopausal, don't eat foods that screw with your sex hormone balance. Even if you are peri-menopausal, skip the soy lobby sound bites and do the research on how hormonally active foods f*ck with your health.

Not going to go into the ethics of humanely raised, grass finished meats, pastured eggs, sustainable seafood, and organic produce here. There's better books and studies out there on the subject.

I know you're excited to see bacon on here (nature's meat candy). But be sure to use it as more of a condiment/flavor-enhancer than an entrée. Ensure that your bacon is pastured and organic. It's more fat than protein so any unclean bacon source will be highly toxic and inflammatory. Besides, pigs are highly intelligent animals that are grotesquely mistreated in the industrial pork factories. Especially the overbred females. It is a no-win for the consumer, the animal or the earth.

VEGGIES
Organic when possible.

- cilantro
- bok choy
- brussel sprouts
- fennel
- celery
- asparagus
- broccoli
- cauliflower
- cucumber
- avocado
- kale (always cooked)
- collard greens (always cooked)
- spinach
- cabbage
- radishes
- summer squash
- zucchini
- lettuce
- green onion
- onions
- shallots
- garlic

OILS & FATS
Let's go over them one more time.
- MCT Oil
- Unrefined, Virgin Coconut Oil
- Grass-fed Organic Ghee
- Grass-Fed Organic Buttter (raw if possible)
- Organic Red Palm Oil
- Free-range, pastured, organic egg yolks
- Grass-fed red meat fat and marrow
- Avocado Oil (do not cook with)
- Macadamia nut oil (do not cook with)
- Cocoa butter
- Chocolate (at least 70% cacao content)

- Organic Extra Virgin Olive Oil (do not cook with)

Due to hydrogenation and partial hydrogenation (see pg. 12), avoid:
Canola oil, corn oils, safflower oils, soy oils, and vegetable oils. Read labels.
Ask questions at restaurants. This stuff sneaks into everything.

Remember, high levels of healthy dietary fat are essential for preserving as much muscle as possible while losing the greatest amount of body fat. The amount of muscle mass you retain is the largest indicator of your resting metabolism. Moreover, it's one of the largest components impacting successful fat loss.

NUTS
Have coconut and olives as much as you want. Consume the rest very sparingly. Remember what we said about Omega-6 PUFA's in the previous chapter? Aside from the coconuts and olives, try to make sure the nuts are raw and sprouted as much as possible.
- Coconuts (wooo hoooo!)
- Olives (yeah!)
- Almonds
- Cashews
- Hazelnuts
- Macadamia
- Pecans
- Chestnuts
- Walnuts

STARCH
We'll be eating these on our carb re-feed days.
- Sweet potato
- Yam
- White rice
- Pumpkin
- Butternut squash
- Taro
- Cassava
- Plantain

I hear you asking, "White rice? I thought brown rice was better for you! WTF?!" White rice and sweet potatoes are lowest in protein toxins. Brown rice and white potatoes are full of mycotoxins, lectins and phytates that bind to vitamins and minerals and prevent them from being absorbed. Remember that leaky gut we talked about earlier? Even if brown rice is higher in nutrients it doesn't matter because they're not being absorbed by your gut.

The reason we do the carb re-feed is for the easily digestible forms of glucose that allow us to keep our fat burning engines on after being in a state of ketosis (adapted to fat burning) for so long.

Here's a study of actual brown rice nutrient absorption from PubMed and The National Institutes of Health: http://www.ncbi.nlm.nih.gov/pubmed/2822877.

FRUIT

Eat sparingly. Fructose is still a sugar. Organic when possible as most of these are heavily sprayed with pesticide. We don't need you sprouting a third arm from your head.

- Cherries (good glucose to fructose ratio)
- Brown bananas (for a glucose spike in protein/smoothies)
- Blackberries
- Cranberries
- Lemon
- Lime
- Raspberry
- Strawberry
- Pineapple
- Blueberries

SWEETENERS

- Stevia (SweetLeaf Stevia is the best, safest brand)
- Raw, Organic Honey (sparingly)

Absolutely NO artificial sweeteners. They actually contribute to weight gain among other alarming health risks. If you want to deep dive into why, research this study and conclude for yourself:

Adverse effects of high-intensity sweeteners on energy intake and weight control in male and obesity-prone female rats. (http://www.ncbi.nlm.nih.gov/pubmed/23398432)

Companies realize the public is cluing into the dangers of artificial sweeteners. Here are some new names they're using to hide these poisons in their products:

TOXIC SWEETENERS TO AVOID

Acesulfame Potassium aka
- ACK
- Ace K
- Equal Spoonful (also + aspartame)
- Sweet One
- Sunnett

Aspartame aka
- APM
- AminoSweet
- Aspartyl-phenylalanine-1-methyl ester
- Canderel
- Equal Classic
- NatraTaste Blue
- NutraSweet

Erythritol

Glycerol aka
- Glycerin
- Glycerine

Glycyrrhizin aka
- Licorice

Neotame

Polydextrose

Saccharin aka
- Acid saccharin
- Equal saccharin
- Necta Sweet
- Sodium saccharin
- Sweet N Low
- Sweet Twin

Sucralose aka
- 1',4,6'-Trichlorogalactosucrose
- Trichlorosucrose
- Equal Sucralose
- NatraTaste Gold
- Splenda

Tagatose

Xylitol

Sneaky bastards. Ok, onto approved spice and everything nice:

<u>SPICES</u>

- Herbs

- Pink salt
- Sea salt
- Pepper
- Ginger
- Apple Cider Vinegar
- Cinnamon
- Coconut Aminos
- Allspice
- Cloves
- Organic mustard

BEVERAGES
- Water and plenty of it (with lemon or lime optional)
- Single blend, wet process coffee
- Premium green tea
- Unsweetened iced tea
- Mineral water
- Club soda

I always try to have soft-boiled eggs and a salad ready made. The crockpot is your best friend. Dump in some meat, veggies, seasoning, voila. On Sundays I will pre-make a lot of food for when I'm on the run during the week. Having food prepared is one way to keep yourself on track, especially after a long day of work (or anything else) when you don't feel like prepping and cooking.

As far as the approved foods go, there are so many amazing recipes you can make, invent and tweak with the above ingredients. Google "paleo recipes" or visit NomNomPaleo.com (http://nomnompaleo.com/post/16824406467/the-whole30-recap-every-single-day) for some Whole 30® approved recipes. There's a full list available in back.

You didn't see red wine or any other spirited libation on the above list because for these initial three weeks, **alcohol is out**.
- It serves no nutritional purpose
- Has twice the amount of empty calories as sugar
- Ages you rapidly
- Gets stored as fat
- Creates chronic systemic inflammation
- Is a neurotoxin that causes you to slur, embarrass yourself and make poor judgments (with food and behavior).
- **It's also worse for women:** Alcohol can increase levels of estrogen and other hormones associated with hormone-receptor-positive breast cancer. Revisit Chapter One

information about alcohol and estrogen if you need a refresher.

If going three weeks without alcohol seems impossible then there are more problems to deal with than your body fat. If you're going out, get a club soda or mineral water with lime. No one will know the difference and you and your wallet will thank me in the morning. We've all been there with alcohol and we'll talk about ways you can minimize its harm in a later chapter. That being said, here is the truth about what you do to yourself with alcohol, even in moderation:

Drinking alcohol almost completely shuts down your body's fat burning ability.
(Siler SQ, Neese RA, Hellerstein MK. De novo lipogenesis, lipid kinetics, and whole-body lipid balances in humans after acute alcohol consumption. Am J ClinNutr. 1999; 70(5):928-36.)

Do not start this program if you can't stop drinking for an extended period. **It will not work, it will backfire and you're wasting your time**. I have a client who followed this program to a tee except for a glass of wine or two at dinner every night and then cocktails over the weekends. Not only did she get a severe case of inflammation ranging from joint and back pain, she also had excruciating foot pain, read: gout, and the weight piled back on. Health is not going to happen when you inject poison into your biome. Time to develop some new habits. Come back when you're serious and dedicated. I'm not here to be your best friend. I'm here to give you your health back. If it's not on the lists above, don't put it in your body.

Additionally, try to drink *at least* three liters to a gallon of water a day. When your body starts becoming adept at burning fat, you're going to need to drink a lot more water. You're also going to be incredibly thirsty as your cells detox and release excess water. The first week or two will be water weight loss and that's a good thing. You'll feel less bloated and know that you're burning up all that excess storage of carbs (glycogen) in order to start hacking away at the body fat for fuel.

This is cool: For every one gram of excess glycogen (stored carbohydrates aka bloat) your body has, it carries with it three grams of water. That can add up to a lot of excess weight (water weight) and is part of the reason you will see a meaningless weight gain after our carb re-feeds. It is not fat, it's water. You can't gain pounds of fat overnight. The higher the stores of carbs and carb consumption you had previously will determine the time it takes your body to become adapted to burning fat. It will also determine the amount of water weight you will lose in the beginning stages. More glycogen stores means more water weight loss initially *for most women* in the beginning. After that, you will start burning actual fat. **I lost ten pounds my first week**. Using my methods, my neighbor (also female, 5'5, 43) lost 16. Transitions can take from as little as one to two weeks up to a month when followed correctly and safely.

When you minimize your carbohydrate intake, your body dips into this excess glycogen for fuel. Each one gram of glycogen begins releasing the additional three grams of water as it's burned. Think about it: a lot of those "problem areas" are fat for sure, but they are also areas where your body stores all the extra carbs you eat that it can't use for fuel initially. These will shrink quickly.

Just as eating a high carbohydrate diet causes you to hold onto water, eating a low-to-moderate carbohydrate diet will act as a diuretic at first. As your cells release all this excess water and detox, you will probably feel dehydrated, hence the need for additional water to flush the garbage out. All these toxins being released by your cells will go through your liver. Let's give that liver a helping hand with ridding the toxins by drinking good, clean water. After all, don't you think we abused it enough in college, at happy hour or possibly last weekend? In a later chapter we're going to go into more ways we can support the liver while it goes into double duty filtering out years of stored toxins.

What about cigarettes? No need to repeat the risks of which you're already aware. Smoking kills women in ways and consistency much different than men, plain and simple. If you smoke, this won't work for you. You cannot simultaneously heal and harm yourself. Decide what's important to you and go from there. Part of this process is cleansing your cells. That can't happen with chosen self-pollution.

More things to expect as you release water weight and cells detoxify:

- You are going to smell and/or have bad breath and possibly increased acne. For a few days I smelled like a boys high school locker room. I was pretty toxic. Keep drinking water. You're probably going to feel like you can't get enough for a few days. We're also going to add mineral-rich pink salt to that water but more on that later.
- Grains, dairy and sugar are addictive just like drugs. Depending on your level of consumption you're going to go through withdrawals. They normally last 4-5 days, sometimes more in extreme cases. Feeling flu-ish, irritable, headache, body ache, lethargy, insomnia are all normal. Eating enough healthy fat and drinking water will help alleviate these symptoms as well as crush the cravings for good.
- Personally, I would not start this program during PMS or your

period if you're prone to insane cravings or mood swings (like I was). There's too much potential for fatigue, failure and beating yourself up when you don't deserve it.

- Expect to see a nice drop in weight. If people try to negate your loss as "it's only water weight," show them the hand (or the finger. Both if it's justified). You have to lose the water weight first before tapping into the fat. It's awesome not to be bloated! Plus, losing that water weight lets you know your body is flipping the switch to fat burning once it rids itself of all those excess carbs.

Here's more good news: once you've finished the ten day carb depletion detox, your skin will look amazing, you'll have less body odor or none, your breath will be fresher, your sleep will be high quality, your energy will stay level, and your hair will be shinier.

Speaking of carbs, let's move on to when we'll be mowing down some safe starches to keep our fat burning engines purring like metabolic Maseratis.

3 HAVE YOUR CARBS AND EAT THEM, TOO
SAFE STARCHES & INSULIN SPIKING FOR FAT LOSS & LEAN MUSCLE GAIN

You can manipulate carbohydrates to create the body YOU want (not the body that magazine covers say you need for acceptance). All this hoopla about "carbs are evil" is crap. It's a blanket, ignorant, unscientific statement to assert that no one should eat carbs ever. For women, it's downright dangerous. Again, you will determine what works best for your unique body. But if you want to keep burning body fat and gain muscle, you must eat some carbs. Commit to it for these three weeks.

Attention recovering sugar addicts: this is not a license to go on a sugar binge. Your diet of healthy fats is going to curb and squash those cravings so the starches we eat going forward will be from the Safe Starch list in chapter two.

REMEMBER: You will most likely see your scale numbers go up after a carb re-feed. If you don't have a body fat measuring tool, try to get yourself tested before you start the program and again after you complete the three weeks. If you have to, keep the scale business down to once a week and don't weigh yourself after a carb re-feed. That's sabotaging yourself.

FACT: Your initial weight loss is going to be water, not fat. We want that. True fat loss takes time and discipline. When you put yourself on a scale you are not measuring actual fat loss. You are measuring fluctuating fluid retention. I did weigh myself almost weekly; however, it was in order to enter the correct overall body weight into my Omron body fat analyzer. The scale number is nothing but a statistic to enter into your bodyfat analyzer. I'm elated when I see my scale number go up and my bodyfat percentage decrease. It means I'm getting stronger and gaining more fat-burning lean muscle! Wooot!

If you do not do a carb re-feed, your fat loss will slow, then plateau and then stop all together. Skipping carb re-feeds is not an option for the truly committed.

WHEN WE EAT CARBS IS CRUCIAL

Maybe you've heard the myth about not eating carbs after 5 p.m. Here's why it's fundamentally flawed regarding fat burning. It's true, muscles are more sensitive to insulin in the morning. That's why "experts" say to have your carbs in the a.m., when they can't be stored as fat. What they fail to mention (or have not researched thoroughly) is that although muscle cells are more sensitive to insulin in the morning, so are fat cells. If you eat your carbs in the morning, a good portion of them will be stored in fat cells.

When done as follows, carb re-feeding is a safe, easy and healthy biohacking strategy that leverages a woman's metabolic rhythm and feeds carbs to your muscles instead of storing them as fat. Losing body fat this way is so simple it's ridiculous. Moreover, it allows cortisol levels to drop because you're not spiking insulin in the morning when cortisol levels are at their highest.

Cortisol's main duty in your body is to break down molecules for fuel. If you do not introduce insulin into your body via carbs in the morning, the complex molecule that cortisol will break down is fat. Keeping insulin out of it will allow you to burn lots more fat. However, once you ingest carbs in the morning (including fruit) and introduce insulin into your system, you've literally screwed your cortisol levels. They skyrocket and turn the tables dramatically from fat burning to fat storing. Throughout the day your cortisol levels will not subside. One of the worst side-effects: a false hunger signal to your brain. Snack much? So, our goal in the morning is to keep insulin levels as low as possible.

DID YOU KNOW? The Curious Case of Corn Flakes

Maybe you're thinking, "If carbs in the morning are so bad, how come almost everyone eats them for breakfast?" From the early 1900's through the 1960's, those in America who could afford it ate mostly high fat proteins for breakfast (eggs, sausage, bacon, ham). The less fortunate ate boiled grains like porridge, gruel, oatmeal, etc.

Enter John Kellog. Yes, of Kellog's Corn Flakes. Besides being a king of boxed, processed carbs, he was also a highly influential physician and Seventh Day Adventist. His healing philosophies at the renowned Battle Creek, Michigan Sanitarium were based on preventing masturbation (he applied pure carbolic acid to the clitorises of women and girls to prevent "onanism"); water and yogurt enemas; and vegetarianism – he believed meat caused sexual arousal. Oh, he was also an active and outspoken racist who helped found The Race Betterment Foundation which sought to breed the superior races of society while sterilizing those deemed "inferior."

Kellogg was the original "celebrity to the stars," tending to many powerful celebrities and politicians of the day. Some of his notable clientele included President William Howard Taft, Thomas Edison, Amelia Earhart, George Bernard Shaw, and Henry Ford.

His influence with these titans of government, industry and celebrity helped evangelize the Kellog Company, their "healthy" corn flakes and many other cheap, carb heavy breakfast staples that still start us off on insulin spikes every day. This is not meant as an affront to Seventh Day Adventism but a point that one wealthy, influential and business-savvy man got the country on board with cheap carbohydrates for breakfast. None of it was based on sound science or nutrition, only religion. Sorry for the sidetrack but I thought you might find that interesting.

Why we eat carbs late in the day. If we keep muscle and fat cells free of insulin in the morning, it maintains your fat burning mode longer throughout the day. We're going to help squash hunger, increase energy, maintain lean muscle, and literally shut your fat cells down with a form of intermittent fasting using MCT oil and grass fed butter coffee. This combo increases your metabolism by 20% without giving you that jittery caffeine feeling thanks to the healthy fats. Plus, it's more delicious than a latte. We'll talk about that in the next chapter. If coffee isn't your thing you can use green tea with a little bit less of a fat burning effect.

Keeping your body in fat burning mode throughout the day also primes your sympathetic nervous system that's responsible for your "flight or fight" response. So, after the ten day carb depletion, you'll do a carb re-feed every three days. These will happen after one of your short, intense workouts. The priming of your sympathetic nervous system will allow you to get maximum effect from your workouts while recruiting more muscle fibers.

Why we carb re-feed after a workout. After your workouts, your muscle cells will be sensitive to insulin because you've worked them so hard for short, intense bursts. In essence, they're ready to receive the glycogen that will make them grow. Meanwhile, the butter coffee will have shut a lot of your fat cells down. So even though insulin sensitivity decreases as the day goes on, your muscle fatiguing workout combined with the intermittent fasting, then high fat/protein/ veggie intake will reverse your muscle cells' insulin resistance. That's when you'll eat your carbs. The insulin uptake feeds your muscle cells, making them grow while preventing the fat cells from receiving anything. Cool trick, huh? And don't worry about the term "fasting." I promise you will not be hungry on this program if you follow it correctly.

On days you carb re-feed:

- First half of the day you eliminate insulin and its nasty side effects by Bulletproof® intermittent fasting with butter coffee and MCT oil. Then eat healthy fat, veggie, and protein meals within an 8 hour feeding window.
- By avoiding insulin for the first half of the day, your body will preferentially burn and release fatty acids. This is good because:
  o You get lean without a calorie deficit because you're still eating fat and protein all day
  o You never feel like you're starving although you've become ketogenic
  o You avoid the adrenal fatigue that happens to a lot of women with plain intermittent fasting.
- When you workout on the day of your carb re-feed, your insulin levels will be lower. This means the releaser for your glycogen stores within your muscle tissues will be adrenaline.
- Because you're a badass and didn't consume carbs for the first half of the day, you'll get a huge spike in adrenaline which is awesome because your muscles are more receptive to adrenaline that breaks down glycogen.
- Adrenaline has to be present for using muscle glycogen, which you will have in hordes. This is why it's typical to see big strength gains immediately.

This is an excellent scientifically- and personally - proven strategy for the greatest success in optimizing your body for fat loss and lean muscle gain. After you workout and have your carb re-feed, your body is primed to store glycogen while you recover overnight. It will load your muscles with nutrients and water which, of course, tightens the skin.

Even better news: Once you flip that switch in teaching your body to burn fat while <u>sticking to the principles</u> that keep you fat adapted, it is actually very hard to gain excess body fat again.

GETTING STARTED: 10 DAY CARB DEPLETION

The hardest part of the program is going to be the first ten days. And it's not even that hard. Ten-day carb depletion is exactly what it sounds like. It is THE critical factor in your fat loss and body detoxification. Repeat it with me: THE CRITICAL FACTOR. It's not an option for those who want to be successful here.

Remember how we talked about burning off the excess glycogen (water weight) and detoxing your cells in the previous chapter? For the first ten days of the program we're going to purge toxins and burn as much of that glycogen and water weight off that we can. We'll be consuming all the healthy fat, protein and vegetables we want as well as intermittent fasting with butter coffee. We're going to be flipping that fat burning switch on for good. Then, on the tenth day, you will do a very short, intense workout in the afternoon and immediately consume safe starches with minimal fat after. It's optimum to do these very short workouts between 3-6p.m.

You can do anything for ten days. If you have a slip up and consume more than 30 grams of carbohydrates (including fruit or alcohol) you'll need to **start all over** or else the program WILL NOT work. That should be a good motivator. Here's a reminder of the safe starches you'll eat on the carb re-feed day:

SAFE STARCHES:
Organic whenever possible, especially sweet potatoes and yams
- White rice
- Sweet potatoes
- Yams
- Pumpkin
- Butternut squash
- Taro
- Cassava
- Plantain

My favorite is a baked sweet potato with pink salt, a honkin' slab of butter and cinnamon. Yum.

WHAT TO DO FOR A CARB RE-FEED
Here's what it looks like.

- **Ten Day Carb Depletion at beginning of the program.**
  - Do your short, intense workouts twice a week, three days apart. More on exercise in chapter five.
  - Butter coffee for breakfast in the mornings as part of 16-18 hours Bulletproof® intermittent fasting (next chapter).
    - For example, if you last ate at 9p.m. last night, wake next morning, drink as much water and butter coffee as you like until 1 p.m. Then, break the fast with healthy fats, protein, veggies. Stop drinking butter coffee by 2 p.m..
    - Eat as much fats, protein, and vegetables from the lists in the previous chapters as you like from 1p.m. to 9p.m.
  - If you cheat and consume any sort of carbohydrates, including alcohol, you <u>must</u> re-start at day one. <u>This is not</u>

<u>optional.</u>

- **On the 10th Day You Carb Re-feed**
  - Plan for your 10th day to be a workout day. Do one of the short workouts detailed in chapter five between 3p.m. and 6 p.m.
  - Include starches from the safe starch list in your post-workout meal or dinner. Keep fat in this meal to a minimum.
  - Keep fruit intake low. Your muscles don't really have a use for fructose.
  - Congratulate yourself on being awesome!

After Day 10 of Carb Depletion
  - You will do the same carb re-feed as instructed above every three days, after one of the short, intense workouts.
  - Continue Bulletproof® intermittent fasting
  - Keep eating healthy fats, proteins, and vegetables after fasting with butter coffee.

Use this program until you reach your desired bodyfat percentage. Give yourself a break every few months for a week or two if you intend to do this for the long term or have a lot of bodyfat to shed. Our bodies are highly adaptable and will always outsmart us if we don't mix things up now and again. Don't go on a bender if you take a break but get out of the routines you've established for a little change. You'll have developed the discipline by that point to return to the program if you need.

One problem with super carb-restricted diets is they can blunt the output of hormones that allow you to burn body fat. By doing a carb re-feed you ensure those fat burning hormones stay ignited for up to five days. Doing your carb re-feed will spike your hormone levels enough to last you until your next refeed.

TOOLS FOR SUCCESS

- Only re-feed with safe starches from the list above. The majority of women cannot get away with consuming transfats and sugars like men.

- Consume high protein on your carb re-feed while keeping fats to a minimum. This is the one night a week you're going to bring your healthy fat intake down so the carbs get absorbed faster.

- Drinking alcohol will not allow you to burn any other calories except those in the booze. Alcohol is a toxin and your body, being the intelligent machine that it is, immediately shifts into overdrive to burn up the poison before absorbing or addressing any other nutrients. Alcohol is a metabolism monkey wrench. It can also impair muscle growth for up to five days after consumption.

- When you sacrifice muscle tissue with unhealthy weight loss habits, alcohol, sugars, and lack of short, intense exercise it slows your metabolism and makes it easier to regain additional body fat.

- People who restrict calories to lose weight sacrifice a pound of muscle for every three-to-four pounds of fat lost.

- It only takes four days of restricting your calories (aka starving yourself) to throw all your major fat burning hormones into complete chaos; essentially shutting their fat burning power down. Food is your friend. Do not fear it. Eat!

- What about vegetarianism/veganism? Tried both myself, including raw veganism. Although I know the intentions behind these diets are mostly honorable, the nutrition is not the same. Yes, many vegetables do contain protein, but plant proteins are incomplete. They are not composed the same as animal protein. In fact, some studies show these diets lead to greater risk of heart disease and stroke from malnutrition. See study here: "*Vegetarianism produces subclinical malnutrition, hyperhomocysteinemia, and atherogenesis*" http://www.ncbi.nlm.nih.gov/pubmed/21872435

- Avoiding animal protein can lead to lower consumption of overall protein and sulfur amino acids. This puts anyone avoiding animal foods at an increased risk of cardiovascular diseases.

- If you are constantly ravenous, that's your body's way of signaling a hormone crash. Take a good look at what you're consuming. Are your meals *at least* 50% fat (outside of carb re-feeds)? Have sugars snuck their way onto your plate? Are you drinking enough water? Getting enough sleep? Are you skipping your two weekly, high intensity workouts? Twice a week for less than twenty minutes. Could it be any easier? No excuses.

ZEN AND THE ART OF SELF-SABOTAGE

When you start burning body fat, looking fit, and feeling great, the positive reactions will pour in. Heads will turn. Enjoy it. You deserve it. But sometimes, unconsciously, those closest to you can undermine your efforts. If someone in your life is *consciously* undermining your efforts to change for the better, 86 them. They're toxic. Let's don't mince words.

Sometimes the metamorphosis you're achieving forces people to take an honest look at themselves – and they don't like what they see. This can project on to you in many ways that send you a hundred steps back:

- "Try some, it won't hurt!"
- "You're too _____ now" ← Anyone who tries to shame you or your body can take a leap.
- When you're drinking buddies say, "You're no fun anymore."

That one's my favorite. If the only way you can enjoy your friends/social situations, and vice versa, is with alcohol, then get new friends and hobbies. Remember, you are responsible for your choices and behaviors. No matter what. You choose the actions, you choose the consequences. Nobody pays for self-abuse but you. Other ways you can sabotage fat loss:

- Consuming alcohol, sugar, gluten, unsafe grains, carbohydrates, too much fruit, soy, dairy
- Eating carbohydrates in the morning
- Skipping carb re-feeds
- Restricting calories
- Doing carb re-feeds too close together
- Eating too much fat on a carb re-feed day
- Not eating enough fat on low-carb days
- Consuming diet drinks, sodas, fruit juices, and artificial sweeteners
- Too much chronic cardio
- **Toxic people who don't value their health or yours.**

What about special occasions?

Here's some great news. On special occasions – and special occasion does not mean Saturday night or Flag Day – allow yourself a little extra. Schedule your carb re-feed night so you can have a piece of that birthday or wedding cake. Make sure you do a quick, high intensity workout earlier in the day and the day after. We're talking a few times a year. Eating crap is still eating crap but that's how you can mitigate the effects without too much stalling of your upwards trajectory.

4 INTERMITTENT FASTING & BUTTER COFFEE
THE HOLY GRAIL OF LOSING FAT & INCREASING MENTAL FOCUS

Do you know what the number one source of antioxidants in America is? Coffee. It's also an anti-inflammatory and thermogenic substance which means, on its own without the cream, sugar, and sweet chemical cancer powders, increases fat loss. So what happens when you add delicious grassfed butter and coconut oil or MCT oil to your cuppa joe? You get a powerful fat burning, brain-boosting concoction that's tastier than a latte and keeps you fuller longer.

Guess what else? Bulletproof® Intermittent Fasting (BPIF) also gives your liver a chance to rest and efficiently eradicate toxins. Our bodies did not evolve to be in a constant state of digestion. It's very recent in human history that so many people have the luxury of walking around snacking and eating all the time. It's taxing on your whole system, especially your liver and gut lining.

Bulletproof® Coffee – The Silver Bullet
You may have heard about butter coffee and butter tea as a recent fad. Hot butter drinks have actually been a staple of Tibetan, Indian and Southwest Chinese cultures since the 10th century. The butter and caffeine provide high caloric energy for nomadic peoples and those who labor at high altitudes like Sherpas. This is where Dave Asprey, who patented his own version of Bulletproof® Coffee and corresponding Upgraded™ Self products, first stumbled upon the notion when served yak butter tea on a trip to Tibet.   He claims he "...staggered into a guest house from the -10 degree weather and was literally rejuvenated by a creamy cup of yak butter tea."

Robb Wolf, author of *The Paleo Soultion – The Original Human Diet*, has also been credited for suggesting grassfed butter in coffee in lieu of breakfast. Regardless of who "invented" it, butter coffee in the morning keeps you burning fat and energized without jitteriness or food cravings.

Dave Asprey did come up with a method of taking his Bulletproof® Coffee to the next level by developing his own unique take on intermittent fasting called (surprise) Bulletproof® Intermittent Fasting (BPIF). This version of Intermittent Fasting is optimal for women, especially those who suffer PCOS, endometriosis, adrenal fatigue, thyroid, and fertility issues. What I really appreciate about Dave Asprey's work is that he takes women's health and nutrition issues seriously. He understands that you cannot blindly apply so many of the widely accepted paleo principles to women as you can to men. He even co-authored *The Better Baby Book* with his wife, Dr. Lana Asprey, from their experience helping her recover from PCOS and infertility over forty. Dr. Lana Asprey is a Karolinska-trained physician who runs an international natural fertility and healthy pregnancy consulting practice. They understand the importance of considering a woman's biochemistry when it comes to optimum health and fat loss.

When I added BPIF into my fat burning arsenal, everything changed almost instantly. And it wasn't hard. Literally, bodyfat started melting with minimal effort. My strength gains soared by cutting my workouts down from an hour a day to an *hour a month*. It's not snake oil. It's science. Follow what I lay out for you here and let your body show you the results.

Fasting sounds like starving yourself! There's a difference between Bulletproof® Intermittent Fasting (BPIF) and outright fasting. BPIF is ketogenic fasting. You are consuming calories (butter and MCT or coconut oil) but keeping your body in a state of ketosis by not consuming proteins or sugars for breakfast. With BPIF you're eliminating insulin spikes and all the havoc it wreaks on your body. Like we talked about in the previous chapter, when you have a butter coffee or another butter drink for breakfast, your body is going to preferentially burn and release fatty acids. You lean out quickly without depriving your body of calories. There's no starvation stage as in regular intermittent fasting.

Here's what BulletProof® Intermittent Fasting looks like:
- o Butter coffee for breakfast in the mornings as part of 16 - 18 hours of Bulletproof® intermittent fasting
  - ▪ Stop eating at 9p.m.
  - ▪ The next morning drink as much water and butter coffee as you like until 1 p.m. Then, break the fast with healthy fats, protein, veggies.
  - ▪ Completely stop drinking butter coffee by 2p.m. (so you can sleep) or have Bulletproof® Upgraded™ Decaf Coffee.

- Although I buy my own wet-processed, single blend caffeinated coffee beans, if you're going to drink decaf buy the Bulletproof® kind because most companies use lesser quality beans and toxic chemicals for decaf.
- Eat as much fats, protein, and vegetables from the lists in the previous chapters as you like from 1p.m. to 9p.m.

That's a total of **eight hours** to eat all the healthy fats, protein and veggies you want. Starvation has no place here.

The Official Bulletproof® Coffee Recipe

- Brew 1 cup (8 oz.) of coffee using filtered water, just off the boil, with 2 1/2 heaping tablespoons freshly ground Bulletproof® Upgraded™ Coffee Beans. (French Press or Clever Cone is easiest)
- Add in 1-2 tablespoons Bulletproof® Upgraded™ MCT Oil™ to the hot coffee (It's STRONG – start with 1 tsp. and work up over several days).
- Add 1-2 tablespoons grass-fed, unsalted butter or ghee
- Mix it all in a blender for 20-30 seconds until it is frothy like a foamy latte

The reason Dave Asprey recommends his coffee beans – besides the obvious – is because of mycotoxin issues in lesser quality beans. I know his beans are very high quality and delicious but many good coffee producers know how to eliminate mycotoxin issues with wet processing. I personally use single blend, wet processed beans from Verve Coffee Roasters (http://www.vervecoffeeroasters.com). If you are going to go the decaf route, I do recommend the Bulletproof® Upgraded™ Decaf Coffee Beans.

Coconut oil contains only 15% medium chain triglycerides (MCT). That's why MCT oil is your optimum choice here. It's six times stronger than coconut oil for fat loss. Interestingly, when the American Soy Association became politically powerful in the 1950's, it began a propaganda campaign of cholesterol phobia related to coconut oil and other competitive products. Contrary to soy's smear campaign, coconut oil does not raise cholesterol nor does it even contain cholesterol. The soy magnates were just pushing to replace coconut in our diets with soy and it worked. Soy is actually a hormone disrupting anti-nutrient as discussed in previous chapters. Women have been marketing victims to the soy lobby for too long.

There are a ton of high quality, pricier products available on The

Bulletproof® Exec's Upgradedself.com site. The ones I use regularly are the Upgraded™ MCT Oil™, Upgraded™ Whey Protein, and Upgraded™ Collagen. Again, I have absolutely no affiliation with any of the products or people mentioned in this book.

Other Butter Coffee/Drink Variations:
- I add Sweetleaf (www.sweetleaf.com) stevia to my coffee
- Add a dash of cinnamon
- Replace MCT Oil with coconut oil. You don't get as much of the thermogenic effect but it still works and is much less expensive.
- Use green tea
- Add ground vanilla bean to the ground coffee
- Try Bulletproof® Cacao Tea
- Try Choffy (www.drinkchoffy.com)

Turning off the starvation signal. Butter coffee/Bulletproof® coffee is excellent at curbing cravings for our food addictions. It's pretty amazing what a profound effect on energy, focus and fat loss a tiny set of changes to a beverage most of us drink daily can have.

If you have +/- 60 pounds of fat (not weight) to lose, most likely your gut health is compromised. The good news is that the butyric acid in the grassfed butter you put in your coffee helps heal your gut lining and decrease brain inflammation. This means your body can actually absorb the nutrients you ingest, helping you to feel fuller and nourished.

If you eat a typical American breakfast consisting of cereals, bagels, fruits, muffins, your liver gets bombarded with fructose from fruits and/or anti-nutrients from grains. Your liver screams, "Bloody hell! Now I'm a chemical factory who has to break this crap down! Damn you!" Your liver blocks you on Facebook and writes snarky comments on the Internet about you. Your liver needs fuel to break down all the junk you've jammed in there. There are two fuels it can use: fat or sugar. Isn't this what most of us want when cravings hit us? Fat or sugar or both? When those cravings hit, it's your poor, overworked liver going into overdrive to get you healthy. The more toxic your body is from sugars and unhealthy fats, the stronger those cravings are. So, what we're doing here with the butter coffee is training your body to rely on fat as a fuel source by keeping protein and starches away from your first "meal" of the day which is butter coffee. We're going to show our livers we love them by not drowning them in alcohol, sugars and anti-nutrients, but supplying it with good ol' healthy fats. Then you break the butter coffee fast with moderate amounts of clean proteins; healthy, pesticide-free veggies and anti-inflammatory fats. All of a sudden, your body awakens. Drink butter coffee for breakfast and blunt those food cravings and crashes for the rest of the day. You become a focused, energetic, fat burning fox. Your liver and skin will re-friend you on Facebook.

What if Bulletproof® Intermittent Fasting doesn't work for me? If you have significant amounts of body fat to lose but the belt loops are still snug, you're more than likely leptin resistant. Leptin is a hormone that is the wizard behind the curtain of everything that happens in your body regarding your weight, thyroid, stress levels, brain function/mental focus, inflammation, reproduction, and heart health. It's the VIP of hormones manufactured in your fat tissue stores. When leptin leaves your fat it hitches a ride in your bloodstream up to your brain, letting your gray matter know how much fuel (fat and sugar) and quality nutrition you have to keep the engine running. With that handy bit of info, your brain decides how fast or slow to run your metabolism, among other things.

Ever been in a car where the needle in the gas gauge gets stuck regardless of how full or empty the fuel tank is? If you have significant amounts of bodyfat, **your gas gauge is stuck**. In women with healthy bodyfat percentages, when leptin tells your brain that fuel reserves are low, you feel hunger and you fill the tank. When leptin tells your brain the tank is full, your brain gives your body permission to hit the gas pedal and drive over the speed limit by cranking up your metabolism and burning up that fuel reserve. When leptin tells your brain the fuel reserves are dangerously low, the brain immediately thinks "famine!" and hits the brakes to conserve fuel. When you carry excess bodyfat and your fuel gauge is stuck, your brain has no idea what's truly in your tank. Most people tend to heed their body's "full" signals when eating aka filling the tank. When you have excess fat, you override that signal for psychological and physiological reasons and begin eating compulsively and emotionally, long after your tanks have been filled twice over. Your leptin has no idea what message to give your brain. For women hovering around obesity, this results in even more rapid fat gain. It becomes a runaway train. Your gas gauge no longer works so your full signal either never comes on or comes on way too late.

Let's get that needle unstuck. This is only for women in the obese category (32%+ body fat). Within thirty minutes of waking, make your butter coffee, but I want you to add about 30 grams of protein. You can:
- Blend in raw egg yolks (delicious) to your coffee
- Eat a few soft boiled eggs (always eat yolks runny or soft)
- Add Upgraded™ Collagen Protein (great for hair, skin, nails, bone density, and lacking in standard American diet)
  - Only use collagen protein in hot coffee
  - Blend in last so as not to "whack" the collagen with blender blades and ruin their protein profile.
- Contrarily, only use whey protein in iced coffee. Like collagen,

add and blend last to preserve protein profile. Hot liquids destroy whey protein.

For all of us with a lot of bodyfat (60+ pounds of fat – not weight) to lose, you may want to do your butter coffee this way for up to three months to firmly establish yourself on a fat loss path. This will ensure you've gotten your body's fuel gauge fixed for good. You're still having fat, you're still having protein but no sugar. Your body will now *prefer* fat as fuel, making gaining back bodyfat more difficult. Once you've become adapted to burning fat, continue with just regular butter coffee without the added protein until you reach your goal body fat percentage.

Food no longer dictates your life. After the first ten days of recalibrating your hormones, healing your gut, eating healthy fats, and letting your liver detox you'll notice something besides a tighter body:

Hunger has no hold on you.

You've kept your body burning the right fuels all day long. A lot of times I only eat twice a day: after I break the fast around one p.m. and then another meal before bed. Sometimes I even have to remind myself to eat. And guess what? It's ok to have all your calories in the evening. Rock a grassfed ribeye and cauliflower mashed "potatoes" drenched in butter. Make sure healthy fat is *at least* 50% of your daily nutritional intake.

Keep your snacking to minimum. If you notice you get hungry before breaking your fast, try adding extra butter to your coffee next time. Snacking is more of an emotional and psychological habit than true hunger. If you're really hungry before breaking your fast, add protein as directed into your second butter coffee drink. This will make you hungrier a couple hours earlier than normal, but that's okay. Humans did not evolve to snack or walk around with a bag of Hershey's kisses and granola bars in their pockets and desk drawers. Really check in with yourself when you start grazing between meals. Is it emotional/psychological craving? Boredom? Habit? Drink a glass of water. Wait twenty minutes. If you feel *truly* hungry after, break your fast and eat some fat, protein and veggies. But understand the difference between hunger and craving first. Hunger is a primal survival signal. Craving is a psychological game.

Now that we've got diet down, let's talk about breaking a sweat no more than twice a week. Your hamster-on-the-treadmill days are over.

5 LOSE MORE FAT, GAIN LEAN MUSCLE WITH LESS EXERCISE
CHRONIC CARDIO STALLS FAT LOSS, EATS MUSCLE TISSUE AND FATIGUES YOUR ADRENALS. STOP IT.

If all you do is diet in an effort to lower a scale number, more than 30% of the weight you lose could be muscle. Diet doesn't do it alone. Not exercising? Not an option.

But here's the good news: you can **burn up to three times more body fat** by cutting your exercise down from an hour a day to simply **two hours a month**. You don't need a gym but you do need to push yourself. Hard. It's not some late night infomercial promise, it's a fact. Short busts of high intensity exercise combined with this nutrition plan catapults your body into a fat burning, muscle growing state.

Here's what you never have to suffer again: chronic cardio. By chronic cardio I mean endurance activities like distance running, treadmill hamstering, elliptical machines, cycling, aerobics. These can be just as detrimental to your health as filling your face full of Cheetos on a non-stop *Orange is the New Black* binge. Chronic cardio, also referred to as steady state cardio, fatigues the immune system. It eats away at muscle (look at a marathoner compared to a sprinter). It raises stress hormone levels like cortisol that can actually signal your body to hold onto fat or store it. And worst of all, chronic cardio can be one of the deadliest things you can do to your heart. Ever hear about dedicated "healthy" runners who have heart attacks out of the blue? Ever notice how distance runners look emaciated while sprinters look strong, toned and tight? Training explosively in short bursts like sprinters, instead of pounding the pavement away forever like cross country runners ignites fat stores, increases growth hormone (a key to anti-aging), and helps teach your body to burn fat for fuel up to 48 hours after exercise. Also, a great side effect of growth hormone is glowing skin!

What we are going to do is something called High Intensity Interval Training (HIIT), twice a week for 8-20 minutes. That's it. It takes little to no equipment, except maybe some running shoes and a kettlebell if you choose. Remember, our goal here is to burn off unhealthy body fat while maintaining muscle – and hopefully gaining more of it in the process. Once you've reached your desired body fat and want to add on more muscle, your diet, carb intake and exercise regimen will be tweaked slightly. We're not going to get into muscle gaining here but if you do have questions, feel free to use the contact info I provided in the intro. Again, I'm not writing this all down so I can run some marketing gimmick and charge you for the pleasure of an email exchange. Send me your questions and I'll do my best to get back to you as soon as I can.

We talked before about the difference between losing fat and losing weight. You could lose a bunch of weight but still have high body fat and flabby areas (aka skinny fat) because you sacrificed precious muscle in order to reach an arbitrary scale number.

Remember: To get a tight, toned, strong physique **you must preserve muscle while burning fat.** Google "skinny fat images" to get the picture. If you're skinny fat you're not much healthier than someone struggling with obesity.

All it takes are tiny but powerful changes to the way you move your body and nourish it. Remember what we said about the Minimal Effective Dose? Here are four short – but incredibly intense – workouts.

Helpful hint: A great timer app for doing all these workouts is Seconds Pro by Runloop.

After the following explanations of the exercises is a step-by-step guide to the workouts.

1. KETTLEBELLS: The Best Kept Fat-Loss Secret

I first read about Tracy "Queen of The Kettlebell" Reifkind's story in Tim Ferris' *The 4-Hour Body*. At 41 and 250 pounds, Tracy discovered kettlebell swinging and a whole foods diet. Then, something amazing happened: She lost 120 pounds, dropping from a size 24 to size 6. I immediately bought a 35lb kettlebell, her DVD *Programming the Kettlebell Swing* and her book *The Swing*. I highly recommend them both.

The kettlebell swing is so potent because it combines strength and cardio in one powerful movement that works almost every muscle in your body. Tracy's kettlebell workout listed at the end of this chapter is only 15 minutes but it's going to be the most ass-kicking, exhilarating 15 minute workout you ever had. It's one of her "On The Minute" workouts. After about four sessions of swinging, you should expect to see some serious tightening and toning all over.

The cool thing about the two-handed kettlebell swing is that it's a very natural, functional movement for your body. It's uncomplicated and just about anyone can do it. Tracy suggests starting with a 20lb kettlebell that you can get at any sporting goods store. I do highly suggest you purchase either one of her instructional DVD's or book, *The Swing*, so you can properly learn the movement for safety and maximum results.

2. HIIT SPRINTS: Get to the Finish Line of Fat Loss

It's very simple. Give your absolute maximum effort for thirty seconds (high intensity) and active rest (low intensity) for ninety seconds. For some of you, this might be a full-out thirty-second sprint followed by a slow jog for ninety seconds. For others who are just getting into exercise, it may be a thirty second power-walk followed by a slower-paced walk for a minute and a half. Regardless, by maximum effort I mean you should be panting hard after your thirty second high intensity interval. This is only **four minutes** of intensely pushing yourself as hard as your fitness level allows with a minute and a half break in between. Anyone can work hard for four minutes.

Do not do this on a treadmill It takes too long to increase/decrease speed. All you need are running shoes and a stopwatch or timer app. Before doing HIIT sprints, be sure to do a proper dynamic stretching warm up for five minutes. Here's a great tutorial for dynamic stretching: http://www.runnersworld.com/stretching/a-dynamic-routine

HIIT Sprints are hardly easy but they help you lose fat and maintain muscle in a very short amount of time.

3. CINDY, QUEEN OF THE COMPOUND MOVEMENT: A Basic CrossFit® Full Body Fat Blaster Muscle Builder

These are functional, basic bodyweight movements that not many women can perform without assistance. Push ups, pull ups, air squats. Just you moving you. There's no use curling little dumbbells if you can't move your own bodyweight. It's not going to be easy but it will be a great way for you to gauge your overall strength and fitness gains. This is the longest workout in your fat blasting arsenal, coming in at twenty minutes. Simple, but not easy.

This workout is as many rounds as possible in twenty minutes of five pull ups, ten push ups and 15 air squats. Keep a record of how many rounds you can do now and compare it in a couple weeks. Then, let me know so I can pat you on the back! You'll be amazed.

If you can't do a full push up, use resistance bands for assistance or, less desirable, do them on your knees. You can Google how to use a resistance band for pushup and pullup support.

Most of us can't do a pull up without assistance, but I promise if you stick with it, you'll be blown away at how strong you become in such a short amount of time. I went from not being able to do a pushup or pullup and using bands and support to knocking out this workout solely on my own for twenty minutes.

This is a workout you can do just about anywhere, which makes it great for travel. It works your whole body, as these movements are the cornerstone of total body strength. If you don't have monkey bars or something nearby you can use for pull ups, purchase an inexpensive doorway pullup bar or rings on Amazon and get some resistance bands – I like Rubberbanditz – to help you with your pushups and pull ups till you're pumping them out on your own!

4. TABATA: Eight Minutes of Exquisite Agony

Yep. That's it. Only eight minutes. The longest eight minutes of your life. Tabata is a form of HIIT training discovered by Japanese scientist Dr. Izumi Tabata and a team of researchers from the National Institute of Fitness and Sports in Tokyo. Simple, effective and can be done anywhere:

- 20 seconds of push-ups
- followed by a 10-second rest period
- then 20 seconds of squats;
- and another 10-second rest.

Alternating between the two moves, you will do eight rounds of each exercise.

Sample exercise schedule. Pick two for your twice weekly workout and change them up as you go. For example:

Week One
Monday Workout: Kettlebell Swings
Friday Workout: Crossfit® Cindy Workout (Push Ups, Pull Ups, Air Squats)

Week Two
Monday Workout: HIIT sprints
Friday Workout: Tabata

Mix 'em up as you see fit. These workouts are a fat-burning, body shaping arsenal that take no time at all. Get after it!

STEP BY STEP WORKOUT GUIDE TO THE FOUR FAT BURNER WORKOUTS:

Although all of these workouts are very short they are incredibly powerful. By go all out, I mean you should have nothing left in the gas tank when it's over.

Begin these workouts when you begin your 10 Day Carb Depletion. Once the ten days are up, schedule your two carb re-feed nights on the same day as your workouts. Mix and match the workouts below to keep things interesting and most of all, effective. Don't do the same workout twice in one week.

WORKOUT #1: TRACY REIFKIND'S TWO-HANDED KETTLEBELL ON-THE-MINUTE WORKOUT

Time: 15 minutes
Keep a record of how many seconds it takes you to swing the kettlebell ten times. Your fitness goal is to complete ten swings in 15 seconds and rest for 45.

Directions: Set a timer for 15 minutes. At the beginning of every minute you will perform a set of 10 swings. Rest until the next minute begins. The faster you go, the more rest you get.

Ten, two-handed kettlebell swings every minute on the minute for 15 minutes.
- 1:00 – Ten swings, rest until minute number:
- 2:00 – Ten swings, rest until minute number:
- 3:00, etc for 15 minutes.

WORKOUT #2: HIIT SPRINTS

Time: 18 minutes and 30 seconds

Directions: Use a stopwatch or Seconds Pro timer app. Warm up with dynamic stretching for four minutes. Go as hard as you can depending on your fitness level for 30 seconds. Actively rest by walking or jogging for 90 seconds. Repeat for eight intervals. Remember, you are only working hard for four of the 18 and a half minutes. Don't cheat yourself. Walk slowly on the low intensity intervals if you need to recover but don't stop moving. This can also be done on a stationary bike or rower machine.

- 4:00 min Dynamic Stretching Warm Up
1. 0:30 High Intensity (sprint, run, or walk)
2. 1:30 Low Intensity (jog or walk)
3. 0:30 High Intensity (sprint, run, or walk)
4. 1:30 Low Intensity (jog or walk)
5. 0:30 High Intensity (sprint, run, or walk)
6. 1:30 Low Intensity (jog or walk)
7. 0:30 High Intensity (sprint, run, or walk)
8. 1:30 Low Intensity (jog or walk)
9. 0:30 High Intensity (sprint, run, or walk)
10. 1:30 Low Intensity (jog or walk)
11. 0:30 High Intensity (sprint, run, or walk)
12. 1:30 Low Intensity (jog or walk)
13. 0:30 High Intensity (sprint, run, or walk)
14. 1:30 Low Intensity (jog or walk)
15. 0:30 High Intensity (sprint, run, or walk)
- Cool down/stretch

WORKOUT #3: CINDY®, QUEEN OF THE COMPOUND MOVEMENT

Time: 20 minutes

Directions: Do a dynamic stretching warm up. Use resistance bands for push ups and pull ups if needed. Can be modified to do pushups on knees but try to use bands instead to maintain proper form. Set a timer for 20 minutes and do as many rounds as possible, in this order:

- 5 pull ups
- 10 push ups
- 15 air squats

Track your progress. Keep a record of how many rounds you do!

WORKOUT #4: TABATA

Time: 8 minutes

Directions: 20 seconds of push ups followed by 10 seconds of rest, then 20 seconds of air squats, followed by another 10 seconds of rest. Alternate between the two exercises so you complete 8 rounds of each exercise.
Program this workout using the Seconds Pro app. 3:00 min dynamic stretching warm up.

1. 0:20 Push ups
2. 0:10 Rest
3. 0:20 Air Squats
4. 0:10 Rest
5. 0:20 Push ups
6. 0:10 Rest
7. 0:20 Air Squats
8. 0:10 Rest
9. 0:20 Push ups
10. 0:10 Rest
11. 0:20 Air Squat
12. 0:10 Rest
13. 0:20 Push ups
14. 0:10 Rest
15. 0:20 Air squat
16. 0:10 Rest
17. 0:20 Push ups
18. 0:10 Rest
19. 0:20 Air Squat
20. 0:10 Rest
21. 0:20 Push ups
22. 0:10 Rest
23. 0:20 Air Squat
24. 0:10 Rest
25. 0:20 Push ups
26. 0:10 Rest
27. 0:20 Air Squat
28. 0:10 Rest
29. 0:20 Push ups
30. 0:10 Rest
31. 0:20 Air Squat
• Cool down

Eight minutes sounds like nothing but depending on your fitness level, you may need to add more rest time. Alternatively, if the squats are easy, try doing goblet squats holding a kettlebell or dumbbell or doing thrusters (combo squat with shoulder press) with dumbbells. If you cannot yet do a full pushup use a resistance band or do them from your knees. Keep your buttcheeks squeezed and belly pulled in tight.

Don't cheat yourself on the high intensity intervals of these workouts. That's where the seeds of muscle growth and fat burn are sown.

Let's put the program all together on the next page.

6 PUTTING THE PROGRAM TOGETHER
SAMPLE SCHEDULE PLANS

CARB DEPLETION PHASE: Days one through ten.
The night before beginning the No Fail Fat Burning for Women® program, stop eating at 9:00 pm. This will allow for a 16 hour ketogenic fasting phase. Adjust the times to your schedule accordingly. Just be sure to allow for a 16 hour fasting phase followed by an eight hour feeding window.

Try to begin on a Saturday (or whenever you have time off). This way, you're not rushed or stressed from work and can prepare your foods while easing into the program. Try to have one day a week where you prep some staple foods like salads, veggies, meats, soft boiled eggs, etc ahead of time. Preparation = success and makes it harder to opt for crap food that sends you back to day one. We go into greater detail of vitamins/supplements most women's diets lack in chapter eight. They are nice-to-haves.

◆ = Workout day. Choose from one of the four workouts in the previous chapter. Don't repeat the same work out twice in one week.

✔ = Carb re-feed day. Eat your safe starches in the evening with a little less fat.

- Night before Day One. Finish eating before 9:00pm.
- ◆**Day 1 (workout day):**
  - ○ Wake, take soil-based probiotic, vitamins D3 & K2, drink butter coffee or butter tea until 1:00pm
  - ○ 11:00 am two-to-five caps of activated charcoal with 8oz. water, away from medications and food
  - ○ 1:00pm – 5:00pm Eat fat, veggies and protein

54

- o ◆Workout between 3:00 and 6:00 pm◆
- o Take other vitamins and supplements if you wish
- o 5:00 pm – 9:00pm Eat fat, veggies and protein

- **Days 2-4:**
  - o Wake, take soil-based probiotic, vitamins D3 & K2, drink butter coffee or butter tea until 1:00pm
  - o 11:00 am two-to-five caps of activated charcoal with 8oz. water, away from medications and food
  - o 1:00pm – 9:00pm Eat fat, veggies and protein
  - o 5:00 pm Take other vitamins and supplements if you wish

- ◆**Day 5 (workout day):**
  - o Wake, take soil-based probiotic, vitamins D3 & K2, drink butter coffee or butter tea until 1:00pm
  - o 11:00 am two-to-five caps of activated charcoal with 8oz. water, away from medications and food
  - o 1:00pm – 5:00pm Eat fat, veggies and protein
  - o ◆Workout between 3:00 and 6:00 pm◆
  - o Take other vitamins and supplements if you wish
  - o 5:00 pm – 9:00pm Eat fat, veggies and protein

- **Days 6-9:**
  - o Wake, take soil-based probiotic, vitamins D3 & K2, drink butter coffee or butter tea until 1:00pm
  - o 11:00 am two-to-five caps of activated charcoal with 8oz. water, away from medications and food
  - o 1:00pm – 9:00pm Eat fat, veggies and protein
  - o 5:00 pm Take other vitamins and supplements if you wish

- ✔ ◆**Day 10 (workout day)!:** Congratulations! The "hard" part is over!
  - o Wake, take soil-based probiotic, vitamins D3 & K2, drink butter coffee or butter tea until 1:00pm
  - o 11:00 am two-to-five caps of activated charcoal with 8oz. water, away from medications and food
  - o 1:00pm – 5:00pm Eat fat, veggies and protein
  - o ◆Workout between 3:00 and 6:00 pm◆
  - o Take other vitamins and supplements if you wish
  - o ✔ 5:00 pm – 9:00pm **Eat safe starches,** veggies, protein, and a little less fat ✔

When/if you feel very strong cravings this is actually your body letting you know the program is working. Eat a little more healthy fats when those cravings hit and allow your body to detox from your food/substance addictions. You can do anything for ten days.

AFTER CARB DEPLETION PHASE

Perform work outs and carb-refeeds on the same days, with three complete days in between. For example, if you work out and carb re-feed on a Monday, your next workout/re-feed day will be Friday. Those days look like this:

Carb Re-Feed/Workout Days
- o   Wake, take soil-based probiotic, vitamins D3 & K2, drink butter coffee or butter tea until 1:00pm
- o   11:00 am two-to-five caps of activated charcoal with 8oz. water, away from medications and food
- o   1:00pm – 5:00pm Eat fat, veggies and protein
- o   ◆Workout between 3:00 and 6:00pm◆
- o   Take other vitamins and supplements if you wish
- o   ✔ 5:00 pm – 9:00pm Eat safe starches, veggies, protein, and a little less fat ✔

Regular Intermittent Fasting Days
- •   Wake, take soil-based probiotic, vitamins D3 & K2, drink butter coffee or butter tea until 1:00pm
- •   11:00 am two-to-five caps of activated charcoal with 8oz. water, away from medications and food
- •   1:00pm – 9:00pm Eat fat, veggies and protein
- •   5:00 pm Take other vitamins and supplements if you wish

Warning: Do not skip your carb re-feed days thinking it will help burn more fat. Skipping carb re-feeds will actually lead to adrenal fatigue, a fat loss plateau, possible weight gain, and more. Carb re-feeds are where your hormones get re-energized to keep on fat burning.

Resist the urge to over-exercise. Your body will need time to recover and repair from these short but intensely powerful exercises. Although brief, they are incredibly taxing on your system. Going for walks or playing the sports you enjoy are fine. These are considered "active rest."
You will not see desired results from this plan if you ingest carbs until the evening of Day 10 during this phase. If you do, start over at day one.

Let's make it easy and don't put yourself in that situation. Your behavior matters and it's 100% your choice and responsibility for what goes down your gullet.

Now, let's talk about some vitamins and supplements you might want to include in your program.

7 VITAMINS, SUPPLEMENTS AND FUN TOYS

Here's why most of your multi-vitamins suck and could potentially be poisoning you: vitamins used in that volume are usually very poor quality (many cases of high lead, contaminant and byproduct levels) and the doses are not always accurate. Plus, packing all those "vitamins" together can cause adverse reactions or they can cancel each other out. Moreover, the supplement industry is unregulated. If you want to hear horror stories of what goes into a lot of the cheap vitamins and supplements sold at big box stores like WalMart or by "celebrities" selling a private label by slapping their names on it, I suggest you check out the work of former FDA Agent Gary Collins (www.primalpowermethod.com). It is your responsibility to do the due diligence when it comes to what you put inside your body. This especially goes for vitamins and supplements. Heavy metals in herbs from China, sawdust and pharmaceuticals in counterfeit vitamins sold on Amazon… the list goes on. If you are considering taking the vitamins and supplements listed below, visit your local, small business vitamin store, talk to the people who work there and look for brands that have been around a while. Ask them what they would give their kid or best friend. I'll also suggest brands I use but again, do your homework and take complete responsibility for your wellbeing. Sorry to be redundant but I want to mention again that I have no affiliation with any of these brands or products. After much experimenting, these are what work for my biochemistry.

Regardless of how clean you eat now, the nutrition in our meats and produce isn't where it was a hundred years ago. Toxins in the soil, water, air and other contaminants in the food supply effect everything that enters our body. Here are some of the vitamins and supplements I highly recommend specifically for women because of deficiencies in our diets.

Vitamin D3

If you're pregnant or thinking about popping out a DNA ball or two in the future, D3 can make all the difference in fertility and the health of your baby. Side note: Vitamin D3 is actually a hormone and was incorrectly labeled a vitamin upon its discovery in the early 20th century.

Babies born to mothers who are D3 deficient have an increased likelihood of:

- Schizophrenia
- Diabetes
- Low birth weight
- Seizures
- Low bone density

Two-thirds of American women are deficient in D3. Even if you're not interested in contributing to the population, according to Dave Asprey's research for his *Better Baby Book,* women who are D3 deficient are at risk for:

- Bacterial vaginosis
- Infertility
- Gestational diabetes
- Increased rate of C-Section
- Bone loss
- Hormonal imbalance
- Insulin resistance
- Hip fractures
- Suppressed immune systems

What D3 does:

- Reduces breast cancer incidents by up to 50% on 2000IU/day (read the study here: http://onlinelibrary.wiley.com/doi/10.1111/j.1749-6632.1999.tb08728.x/full)
- Increases the absorption of calcium for stronger bones and teeth.
- Destroys pathogens in the body
- Helps alleviate and prevent Polycystic Ovary Syndrome.
- **Exciting:** A recent study shows a high dose of Vitamin D five days before menstruation significantly reduces severe menstrual cramps (Bertone-Johnson E, et al "Vitamin D for menstrual and pain-related disorders in women" *Arch Intern Med* 2012; 172: 367-369.)

The reason why I suggest taking D3 in the morning with your soil-based probiotic is because it literally is the "sunshine" vitamin. You don't want that burst of energy to impact your sleep by taking it later in the day.

For more information on D3 and dosing, visit http://www.vitamindcouncil.org/about-vitamin-d/how-do-i-get-the-vitamin-d-my-body-needs/

Suggested brand: Mega Food D-3 2000IU or Purity Products D3

Vitamin K2
I can't say enough good things about this vitamin. Almost every single woman, and her children, eating a standard American diet is deficient. I suggest taking this in the morning as it works best with Vitamin D3. If you're really interested in the fascinating story and benefits behind K2, read Dr. Kate Rheaume-Bleue's book *Vitamin K2 and The Calcium Paradox: How a Little-Known Vitamin Could Save Your Life.*

Another good reason for eating grass-fed/finished meats and organs, pastured eggs, grassfed butter and COOKED dark, green leafy organic vegetables is because of the K2 content you will not get in industrial foods. It's also highly available in Natto, a type of fermented soybean byproduct. I don't recommend Natto because of the likelihood you're going to get a GMO frankenfood soy product that could outweigh the benefits of K2.

Moreover, for women with children – especially girls – supplementing with K2 can help prevent osteoporosis in their womanhood. Almost all of today's American children are K2 deficient. Supplementing their diets with K2 supports bone development, bone mineral density, and bone strength, and may contribute to the development of their cardiovascular health

Take K2 for:
- **Healing dental cavities and tooth sensitivity** (I swear by this)
- Preventing/reversing osteoporosis and bone fractures
- Preventing plaque in coronary arteries that leads to heart disease (a silent killer of women)
- Regulating calcium to the appropriate places in the body
- Proper blood clotting
- Suppressing liver cancer

Suggested Brand: Life Extension

Vitamin C
Dave Asprey, The Bulletproof Executive™, writes of Vitamin C:

"This is one of the safest, most effective supplements you can take. Vitamin C is needed for collagen and connective tissue formation. It's used to manufacture glutathione, the most powerful antioxidant in the body Vitamin C can enhance immune function and help quench free radical damage. Studies have shown you can take up to 120 grams of vitamin C a day with no side effects (besides loose stool)."

It's hard to get enough vitamin C from food, which is why 30 percent of the population is deficient.

Some fruits and vegetables are high in vitamin C, but cooking and storage methods can deplete vitamin C content. Supplementation with at least 500mg per day is optimal. You should take a lot more if you are suffering from chronic infections or healing from injury.

Forms: Ascorbic acid crystals or time release capsules.

Time Taken: Morning and evening, but it's best not to take it after a workout as isolated antioxidants can negate the insulin sensitivity gained from exercise.

Suggested brand: Solaray

Source: http://www.bulletproofexec.com/optimize-your-supplements/

Fish Oil

Although many people prefer Krill Oil, I absolutely do not agree with the argument that it's a sustainable supplement. I'm not going to get into Mercola studies or those things here, but as a longtime, hardcore ocean advocate I do not recommend Krill Oil. I'll leave that for you and your conscience to decide. What I do recommend for women in optimizing immune function and a healthy heart, among other things, is fish oil.

Don't skimp on fish oils. Find a brand that tests for environmental toxins, dioxins and PCB's. Our oceans are incredibly polluted so only opt for the best here.

Suggested brand: Nordic Naturals Ultimate Omega

Soil-Based Probiotics

Hate to break this to you about your beloved yogurt that's become such a huge industry in America. The beneficial bacteria you think you're getting in industrial-produced yogurt cannot survive your stomach acid. Moreover, it's contributing to your fat gain and/or weight loss plateau. An *International Journal of Obesity* study ((2012) **36,** 817–825; doi:10.1038/ijo.2011.153) found an association between obesity and histamine producing bacteria like

Lactobacillus casei, Lactobacillus reuteri, and Lactobacillus bulgaricus that are commonly found in the majority of yogurts and fermented foods, especially when they are not balanced by other species. Rampant unbalanced focus on lactobacillus in yogurt has led to this problem, along with overuse of antibiotics that wipe out good gut bacteria along with the bad.

The factory-farmed milk used for yogurt today has very little in common with the yogurt-forming milk from healthy cows of yesteryear. Not to mention the sweeteners, sugars, and food dyes that go into these things. Ever wonder what some of the most popular yogurt brands use to make the berries look so red instead of actual fruit? It's called Carmine—a dye extracted from the dried, pulverized bodies of cochineal insects. These bugs are used to give several varieties of fruit-flavored yogurt their color.

I digress. Cows that are fed antibiotics, grains and glutinous grains cause their bodies and their milk to contain unhealthy fats you don't see in sustainably raised grass-fed cows. Read Richard Nikoley's article titled *Probiotics: The Genetic Component of Obesity* on his web site http://freetheanimal.com/2014/02/probiotics-component-obesity.html

A high-quality soil-based probiotic:
- Combats depression
- Clears brain fog, histamine and inflammation
- Increases nutrient absorption in the gut
- Assists fat loss
- Fights bad breath and body odor
- Promotes normal bowel movements
- Maintains Healthy GI-Tract MicroFloral Ecologies
- Helps eliminate acne, eczema and psoriasis
- Fights candida

Why soil based probiotics?

Beneficial soil and plant based microbes used to be ingested as part of food grown in rich, unpolluted soil. However, for the last 50 years we have been sterilizing our soil with pesticides and herbicides, destroying most bacteria both bad and good. Our modern lifestyle, which includes antibiotic drug use, chlorinated water, chemical ingestion, pollution and poor diet, is responsible for eradicating much of the beneficial bacteria in our bodies. A lack of beneficial microbes often results in poor intestinal and immune system health, contributing to a wide range of symptoms and illnesses.

The main component of this type of probiotic is the Homeostatic Soil Organisms (HSOs). The naturally occurring colony of probiotics are non-mutated from the original cultures found in unpolluted soil and plants. The HSOs are in a substrate of nutrient rich superfoods providing vitamins, minerals, trace elements, enzymes and proteins. The probiotics are then made dormant using the Microflora Delivery System, which protects the probiotics and delivers them directly to the GI tract where they multiply and flourish.

How do HSOs Work?

Impervious to stomach acids and the digestive process, the microorganisms move through the stomach to the intestinal tract where they form colonies along the intestinal walls. HSOs multiply in the intestines and actually compete with harmful bacteria and yeasts for receptor sites, crowding out the pathogens and taking up residence. Once established, the organisms quickly begin producing the proper environment to absorb nutrients and help to re-establish the proper pH. According to early research and anecdotal evidence the following is a summary of the actions of HSOs

• HSOs work from the inside of the intestines dislodging accumulated decay on the walls and flushing out waste.

• They break down hydrocarbons, a unique ability to split food into its most basic elements allowing almost total absorption through the digestive system. This increases overall nutrition and enhances cellular development.

• They produce specific proteins that act as antigens, encouraging the immune system to produce huge pools of uncoded antibodies. This increased production of antibodies may significantly boost the body's ability to ward off diseases.

• HSOs are very aggressive against pathological molds, yeasts, fungi, bacteria, parasites and viruses.

• They work in symbiosis with tissue or organ cells to metabolize proteins and eliminate toxic waste.

• They stimulate the body to produce natural alpha-interferon. Alpha interferon is a potent immune system enhancer and a powerful inhibitor of viruses.

• HSOs provide critical Lactoferrin supplementation. The microbes produce lactoferrin as a by-product of their metabolism. Lactoferrin is an iron binding protein essential for retrieving iron from foods.

What's the difference between soil based probiotics and other probiotics?
Even if they manage to get through the destructive stomach acids, most probiotics have a hard time implanting in colons that are pH imbalanced or

have too many harmful bacteria. HSOs are designed to implant in any colonic environment. These probiotics colonize throughout the digestive tract where they get to work. These bacteria thrive on their long journey through the GI tract. Most probiotics on the market today will grow bacteria and then, in a centrifuge, separate them from their substrate.

Since most probiotic supplements contain live cultures, they are temperature and age sensitive; therefore requiring refrigeration. If room temperature can begin to degrade these probiotics, imagine what the warm human body will do. The HSOs are dormant in the caplet and activated by fluids. The Primal Defense soil based probiotic I **strongly** recommend requires no refrigeration.

Soil based probiotics are hardy and designed to resist heat, cold, stomach acid, chlorine, fluorine, ascorbic acid and bile. The efficacy of a probiotic should be based upon the ability of the product to "on ferment" foods.

If you want to test the viability of your current probiotic:

Drop a few caplets in 2-4 ounces of milk and leave at room temperature for 24-48 hours. If the probiotic is viable, the milk will change to a thick yogurt-like consistency. This measures the ability of a probiotic to produce enzymes and break down or pre digest food. If a probiotic cannot pass this simple test, do you think it will be capable of doing it's job in your body?

Highly suggested brand: Garden of Life Primal Defense Ultra. I cannot recommend the power of this probiotic enough. Makes me feel like Wonder Woman combined with K2.

Time taken: In the morning then work up to 3x/day.

Activated Charcoal
This stuff saves my life and liver. You're especially going to need this to expedite detoxification during your ten-day carb depletion. Because it *adsorbs* toxic and foreign substances from your body, you want to take it away from medicine, including birth control. After much trial and error I use only the Bulletproof® Upgraded™ Coconut Charcoal. Here's why your choice of activated charcoal matters.

Time tested for over 10,000 years, activated charcoal is the world's oldest detoxing remedy. For centuries, charcoal has been used in Chinese Medicine, Ayuredic Medicine, and Western Medicine as an adsorbent agent to many poisons and intestinal issues.

Fast Detoxing for Better Digestion & Rejuvenation
*   Adsorbs Toxins That Can Cause Digestive Issues and Brain Fog

- Supports Relief of Gas and Bloating
- Made From Pure Coconut Shells
- Ultra Fine Grain For Maximum Adsorption
- Fully Washed To Remove Heavy Metals

Activated charcoal is a highly absorbent material with millions of tiny pores that can capture, bind, and remove up to 100 times the charcoal's own weight in toxins. Four capsules of Upgraded™ Coconut Charcoal has about the same surface area as a football field, which makes it ideal for removing potentially toxic substances from your digestive tract. The porous surface has a negative electric charge that attracts positively charged unwanted toxins and gas so they can easily leave the body.

Toxins from low quality, processed food, and environmental pollution are a real problem. It is important to help your body eliminate them to promote a healthy digestive system and brain. Chronic exposure to toxins produces cellular damage, allergic reactions, compromised immunity, and more rapid aging. Regular use of activated charcoal is easy on the colon and can remove unwanted toxins from your body, leaving you feeling renewed and more vibrant, often in minutes.

The ultra fine and highly purified Upgraded™ Coconut Charcoal uses acid washing, a more expensive extra step that removes toxic heavy metals that are a problem in many preparations of charcoal. The finer the charcoal grains, the better it works.

Charcoal is proven to bind to mold toxins and many other organic poisons that may be present in the environment and in the body.

Because activated coconut charcoal is mainly used to remove toxins from the body, it is great to use when consuming food of unknown quality, eating out at restaurants, or drinking alcohol. If you are feeling moody or suddenly tired, activated charcoal can act as a detox and get you back in the game faster.

Toxicology studies show activated charcoal to be harmless, not interfering with sleep, appetite, or well-being. Everyone responds differently to different doses, so to avoid potential undesirable effects such as constipation, please consult your doctor and use only as suggested.

Suggested brand: Bulletproof Upgraded™ Coconut Charcoal (upgradedself.com)

Time taken: take two or more capsules when detoxing, consuming food of unknown quality or drinking alcohol.

I believe the above vitamins/supplements are truly essential to a woman's overall health. I know they're severely lacking in our diets. As far as vitamins and supplements go, I don't take a vitamin for something I can get largely from a whole food. Consume nutrient-dense foods first then add vitamins and supplements your body can't manufacture or doesn't receive even in your diet.

OTHER VITAMINS AND SUPPLEMENTS I USE

These are nice-to-haves that work for my biochemistry and athletic regimen.

- Vitamin A
- Vitamin B12
- Magnesium
- Potassium
- L-Glutamine (gut health, wound healing, muscle repair)
- BCAA's (muscle repair and recovery)
- Bragg's Apple Cider Vinegar (detoxing, pH balancing)
- Himalyan Pink Salt (trace minerals, adrenal fatigue)
- Garden of Life Raw Green Superfood (I use this to break my fasts sometimes)
- Bulletproof® Upgraded™ Whey Protein 2.0 (www.upgradedself.com)
- Bulletproof® Upgraded™ Collagen Protein (www.upgradedself.com)
- Bulletproof® Upgraded™ MCT Oil (www.upgradedself.com)
- Bulletproof® Upgraded™ Glutathione Force (www.upgradedself.com) Anti-oxidant, liver support, optimal brain and immune function

Again, the supplements like MCT oil, whey, collagen, glutathione are available on the mass market but I've yet to find those that parallel the Bulletproof® quality. Ultimately your body and bank account will decide what's best. These vitamins and supplements are nice to have but you can also achieve the majority or your fat loss/lean muscle goals through following the plan with clean foods and plenty-o-water.

FUN TOYS!

Here are a few gadgets I keep in my quiver that make healthy living easier on the go.

Clever Coffee Dripper (L)

For about $20, makes an amazing cup of coffee. Better than a French press in my opinion, plus travels easy and minimal clean up. BPA-free. Easy peasy. Available on Amazon and a lot of cool coffee shops full of tattooed and/or pierced hipsters.

Aerolatte®

This makes mornings so much easier and less messier. Instead of making a huge butter coffee mess in the blender, grab an Aerolatte® steam free frother for about $15 at Bed, Bath and Beyond. It's a little hand-held stick that allows you to froth your coffee, butter and oil into a delicious latte the cup. Awesome for travel and no mess.

Omron® Body Fat Loss Monitor model HBF 306-C

As mentioned earlier, our goal is fat loss, not weight necessarily weight loss. For around $25 it gives you a consistent reading via bioelectrical impedance within seven seconds. For a truly accurate body fat analysis you might want to get a hydrostatic underwater weighing that many facilities do in a tank. These run from $60 - $100. Or, stick with the Omron and the mirror to be your guides.

Rubberbanditz

A socially and environmentally conscious resistance band company that sells a plethora of bands and equipment that can aid you with push ups, pull ups and working out while traveling. Prices vary depending on bands. www.rubberbanditz.com

Nayoya Wellness Gymastics Rings

I got a pair of these along with Rubberbanditz resistance bands to increase my upper body strength with pull ups, chin ups and dips. These go for about $35 on Amazon.com and travel easy. Loop them over anything and adjust the length as your exercise calls for. Combined with Rubberbanditz, they're an all-in-one portable powerhouse gym.

8 EXCEPTIONS, TIPS AND TOOLS FOR ACHIEVING YOUR ULTIMATE HEALTH
ADRENAL FATIGUE, ALCOHOL, AUNT FLO & MORE

As you've noticed by now, I'm a little obsessed with being my own guinea pig when it comes to what works best for my health. Here are some neat hacks I've learned along the way.

Kickstart Your Morning Energy & Adrenals With Himalayan Pink Salt

I have a major salt fetish and I'm not talking about that toxic, overly processed iodized, heart attack table salt. That kind of salt *is* the enemy. However, pink salt is one of the purest, most nutrient dense salts available. It's rich in iron, electrolytes and contains over 84 trace minerals that our bodies require but do not get in diet alone. These nutrients give pink salt its hue. What about sea salt? Unfortunately, consider how polluted our oceans are and then add the fact that it's still processed. Sea Salt is a better choice as a condiment than table salt but not much. Pink salt is so much more.

More women suffer from adrenal fatigue and thyroid imbalance than we realize. Salt – specifically pink salt – is a cornerstone to restoring adrenal function. If you are someone who is a salt craver, especially around your menstrual period, that's your body screaming for the trace minerals in pink salt.

To combat fatigue, increase mental focus and jumpstart your adrenals in the morning:

- Dissolve ½ tsp of pink salt in warm water (place by bedside night before for ease)
- Drink while still in bed, before rising
- Slowly work up to 1tsp

- Also a great mid-afternoon pick-me-up
- Helps alleviate PMS symptoms
- Good for post-workout recovery
- Helpful for hangovers

Pink salt combined with a high, healthy fat diet is key for a woman's adrenal health and energy. I use Himalania™ Pink Salt.

When Aunt Flo Comes to Town
(or how to combat PMS and killer cramps)

My uterus and I have had a love/hate (mostly hate) relationship since I was twelve. As a Division I athlete in college my bodyfat dropped so low my period disappeared for four years. It returned with a vengeance when I was no loner working out 4-6 hours a day. Moreover, I thought I was being healthy on a low-fat, high carb diet while avoiding eggs, red meat and drinking tons of industrial skim milk… you know, for bone and heart health. Ugh. My periods were 100% debilitating. I couldn't walk much less go to work. I was diagnosed with endometriosis and polycystic ovary syndrome (PCOS). Doctors urged me at 24 to have a complete hysterectomy. A second opinion from a more "progressive" gyno suggested a laproscopy followed by a medical menopause. Yep! I get to experience menopause twice. Luckily, I have the tools now to embrace it better as I near that stage.

Besides the physical ailments that come along with our periods, there are psychological ones at play. Sometimes depression, brain fog, breast tenderness, radical mood swings, cravings, irritability, and extreme fatigue takeover. The first thing to do is understand that this is not YOU but a biological process of your body. Meditation really helps me with this. There are some excellent guided meditations on iTunes called Meditation Oasis. I also listen to Tara Brach's *Radical Acceptance* podcasts and meditations.

I digress. These symptoms of PMS signaling our pending menstruation are triggered by increased estrogen in our bodies. When it comes down to it, it's basically a regularly scheduled hormone imbalance. Things that make managing the estrogen level worse:

- Sugar
- Dairy
- Alcohol
- Gluten

These are the Four Horsemen of a Homocidal Period. Some research says caffeine contributes to it but not for me. I think it's because I'm not adding pasteurized, hormone-whacking creamer or sugar into my coffee. You be the judge for you.

In addition to avoiding the Four Hoursemen of a Homocidal Period (which you should be doing anyway), here's what will help you become BFF's with your Aunt Flo:

- Increase your Vitamin D3 intake during your first signs of PMS. Get your blood levels tested and check with your doctor about dosage.
- Supplement with Magnesium. Among other things, it reduces the severity of cramps.
- At least 500mg of B-6 daily and **grassfed only** organ meats
- ½ to 1tsp of pink salt in warm water every morning or as fatigue indicates
- Eat more soft boiled or over-easy pastured egg yolks
- Move your body more. If it's not your workout day, choose active resting like a walk or bike ride. Get the lymphatic system moving.
- Add safe starches. This is why I don't want you to start the ten-day carb depletion during PMS or your period. If you're really feeling in the crapper, add the approved safe starches to your meals AT NIGHT. This is not license to gorge but do it until your body feels better.
- Up your fish oils.
- Allow yourself extra sleep.

About Last Night. Or, How to Hack a Hangover

I think I hammered home the point about alcohol already. So here's what do if happy hour turns into crappy hour. This hack is from Dave Asprey of The Bulletproof® Executive. He has a cool infographic on hacking hangovers here: http://www.bulletproofexec.com/alcohol-without-the-hangover bulletproof-partying-business-networking/

This may get you some funny looks at the bar but it's better than feeling like a bag of smashed assholes the next day. Before every drink take:

- Nac-Acetyl Cysteine 600 mg
- Vitamin C 1000mg
- Vitamin B1 100mg
- Alpha Lipoic Acid 250mg

When you're finished drinking take:

- Bulletproof® Upgraded™ Activated Coconut Charcoal

Extra insurance:

- Drink ½ tsp of pink salt in 8oz warm water after alcohol drinking is over
- Take a dose or two of Bulletproof® Upgraded™ Glutathione

Remember, this isn't a license to get plastered. This only helps mitigate *some* of the toxic and anti-aging effects of alcohol.

Alcohols to avoid because of toxic fermentation byproducts (resulting in nastier hangovers):
- White wines
- Red wines
- Dessert wines
- Beer

"Safer" alcohols:
- Vodka
- Gin
- Tequila
- Whiskey
- Other distilled spirits

Obviously, watch the sugary mixers and chemical sweeteners that go into a lot of cocktails. My best bet for boozin'?
- Tito's® Handmade Vodka, club soda, squeeze of lime

Body Odor is The Pits!

Two things you might notice once you've detoxed and eliminated processed foods and sugar from your diet:

1. Your body odor is gone or significantly reduced.
2. You only get body odor when you wear a commercial deodorant.

I'm not going crunchy hippie Earth mama on you, but it's important to note that your skin is your biggest organ. It absorbs environmental toxins as well as the topical toxins like chemically-laden lotions, sunblock and deodorants you apply to its surface. One of your skin's biggest jobs is eliminating toxins via sweat glands.

Besides being endocrine disruptors, the aluminum and parabens in deodorants and anti-perspirants clog sweat glands, preventing the natural removal of toxins. It literally traps the stink in. Eliminating sugars, grains, dairy, and alcohol will go a long way to keep your funk at bay. We don't smell like roses all the time. This is especially depends on hormone balance during the menstrual cycle. Here's a natural deodorant recipe that's simple, cheap and easy to make. A lot of people include baking soda in their deodorants but I find it tends to be an irritant for some. Here's what I do:

In a glass container with a lid mix:
- ¼ cup unrefined liquid Coconut Oil (its antibacterial qualities are great). Leave it in the sun to get it about 76 degrees. This is the temperature where it's no longer solid. You could also substitute MCT oil for coconut oil.

- ¼ cup organic arrowroot starch
- 4tbsp. organic, non-gmo cornstarch
- Add drops of your favorite essential oil as you see fit. I just made a batch with sweet orange essential oil and a little cinnamon powder sprinkled in.

Whisk it all together then let it set in the fridge for twenty minutes. Once set you can keep it in your medicine cabinet. It will last for months. Play around with the recipe. I use a little more of the starches than some recipes because I am outside, active and sweating constantly so I need more absorbency. It goes on clear and does not stain.

I also use coconut oil and/or MCT oil for a moisturizer, wrinkle repair and scars.

How to Get Deep, Quality Sleep

To be successful in this program, you need to make sleep a priority. It's where your body and mind repair and grow.

- Ideally, two hours before bed, turn off "blue light" devices like electronics, computers, phones, etc. Do a digital detox as part of winding down your day. Blue lights emitted from electronics signal to your brain that it's day and drastically disrupt your circadian rhythm.
- Power down other lights in your house as bedtime nears.
- Replace some lights in your bedroom and around your home with red LED lights and turn those on as you get closer to calling it a day. Basically, any other color except red light suppresses the normal nightly production of melatonin.
- Drink a cup of 1-2tbsp Upgraded™ Bulletproof® Collagen Protein, 1tbsp MCT Oil, 8oz warm water.
- Take up to 400 mg Magnesium with 200mg Potassium
- Make your sleeping space electronics free and dark as possible.

The MCT oil is cellular fuel and the collagen protein gives your body the building blocks it needs for repair processes. Sleep is when your body does a ton of fat burning and repairs muscles to come back stronger and shapelier. This is another reason why I have you eat your carbs at night during re-feeds. They will elevate your sleep quality by raising the sugar stored in your liver just enough that your brain has more fuel to go through the night.

Improving sleep quality burns more bodyfat than going to bed on an empty stomach. If you don't have enough energy to fuel your brain for deep sleep, dreaming and making hormones, it will impair fat burning. For more on the science of modern sleep read T.S. Wiley's *Lights Out: Sleep, Sugar and Survival* .

9 HELPFUL RESOURCES

COOKBOOKS/REFERENCE

Make sure to use/substitute foods from the approved lists in some of these recipes

- *Nom Nom Paleo Food for Humans* by Michelle Tam and Henry Fong
- *Well Fed 2: More Paleo Recipes for People Who Love to Eat* by Melissa Joulwan
- *It Starts with Food* by Dallas and Melissa Hartig
- *Upgraded Chef – Cooking the Bulletproof Way* by Dave Asprey
- *The Bulletproof® Diet Book* by Dave Asprey
- *The 4-Hour Body* by Tim Ferriss
- *The Swing!* by Tracy Reifkind
- *Carb Nite® Solution* by John Kiefer
- *Body by Science* by Doug McGuff, M.D., and John Little

PODCASTS

- Paleo for Women: http://www.paleoforwomen.com/our-stories-the-podcast/
- Bulletproof Radio: www.bulletproofexec.com/category/podcasts/
- The Tim Ferriss Show: fourhourworkweek.com/category/the-tim-ferriss-show
- Fat Burning Man with Abel James: http://fatburningman.com/tag/podcast/
- BioJacked Radio: athlete.io/category/biojacked-radio/
- The Paleo Solution Podcast: robbwolf.com/podcast/

WEBSITES

- Bulletproofexec.com

- Nom Nom Paleo's 30 Days of Whole 30™ Recipes. These are mostly ll approved and delicious!
  http://nomnompaleo.com/post/42057515329/the-round-up-30-days-of-whole30-recipes
- Women on the Bulletproof® Diet:
  http://forum.bulletproofexec.com/index.php?/forum/19-women-on-the-bulletproof-diet/
- Amanda Allen's Fit as F*ck Challenge:
  http://amandaallen.com.au/media/

Amanda Allen is one of my personal heroes. Amanda Allen is the 2013 and 2014 Crossfit Games Masters Champion (40-44) and an all around mega-athlete. She found Crossfit when trying to make Worlds in canoeing and after someone told her it would help supplement her abs workout! Before kicking ass at Crossfit, Amanda was a professional Triathlete and Track Cyclist with state, national and world titles in both and even tried her hand at firefighting. She is a Personal Trainer and Lifestyle Coach in Adelaide, Australia, and her dog's name is Pep. She does a "Fit as F*ck" challenge every few months that she says, "This Fit as F*ck challenge brings together everything I have ever learned and developed over 2+ decades as an athlete and woman on a gnarly journey toward Fit As F*ck-ness! This challenge is everything I wish someone could have offered my decades ago when I was suffering and trying I be all that I am today! Embrace it all and step up – time to get some!!!"

She is a true inspiration. Check her out. You'll be better for it. And, finally, I'm leaving you with a very special parting gift. That's right, it's my confidential protein shake recipe I've been keeping under wraps. But since we're such good friends now, I'm going to share it with you.

SKYE ST. JOHN'S KICKASS COCONUT MILK PROTEIN SHAKE!
This tastes like an awesome dessert.

- ¼ can full fat coconut milk
- 1 raw, pastured egg (I use duck eggs in these because they have triple the nutrition)
- If it's a carb reefed day, add a couple pieces of frozen, browned banana. I always have these sliced and in the freezer. If it's a non carb reefed day, use a couple ice cubes and add some stevia
- Cacao powder to taste
- 1 tbsp MCT oil
- Blend thoroughly then…

- Add two scoops of whey protein powder. Remember, we add the proteins last and pulse briefly so as not to damage the protein profile by whacking it repeatedly with the blender blades.
- Sometimes if I have a little leftover butter coffee, I'll throw it in there, too.

Enjoy and go conquer the world!

THE END. GO GET 'EM!

ABOUT THE AUTHOR

Skye St. John is a former NCAA Division One athlete and current surfer, martial artist, writer, researcher, and CrossFitter. Her lifelong passion is seeking, researching and experimenting with the science behind optimum mental and physical performance for women. When not catching waves or lifting heavy weight, Skye helps others realize their athletic and creative potential. She lives in San Francisco but loves traipsing the world looking for the next great wave. Contact Skye at burnbodyfatforwomen@gmail.com. Follow her on Twitter at SkyeStJohn. Instagram: Skye_St_John

ABOUT THE EDITOR

Lisa Mecham is a freelance writer and editor living in Los Angeles. Her work has appeared in various literary magazines and she's served as a contributor to *The Rumpus*, as a reader for Tin House, and on the editorial staff staff of *Origins* and Unboxed Books. She is currently finishing her first screenplay.
More at lisamecham.com